Original French edition:
"Écoute et mange, STOP au contrôle ! "
First printing: 2009.
CAN ISBN 978-2-920932-30-2

Copyright © 2011 by Lise Bourbeau
First edition/First printing
National library of Canada
Bibliothèque et Archives nationales du Québec
ISBN 978-2-920932-34-0

Worldwide distributor
Lotus Brands Inc.
P.O. Box 325
Twin Lakes, WI
53181 USA
Tel: 262-889-8501 or 1-800-824-6396
Fax: 262-889-2461
Email: lotuspress@lotuspress.com
www.lotuspress.com

Publisher
Les Editions E.T.C. Inc.
1102 Boul. La Salette
Saint-Jerome (Quebec)
J5L 2J7   Canada
Tel: 450-431-5336; Fax: 450-431-0991
Email: info@leseditionsetc.com
www.leseditionsetc.com

Printed in Canada

LISE BOURBEAU

BEST-SELLING AUTHOR OF
"LISTEN TO YOUR BODY, your best friend on Earth"

Just listen
to your body
and eat

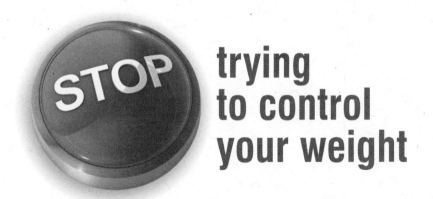 trying
to control
your weight

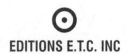

EDITIONS E.T.C. INC

Table of Contents

Acknowledgments

It is very difficult for me to thank only a few of those who helped bring the idea for this book to fruition. My passion for this subject has led me to more than thirty years of research on it. I have gathered testimonies from countless individuals, whom I encountered in my professional as well as my personal life. They come from various countries and cultures and every age group.

I have documented several sources and have, in particular, synthesized my own personal experiences along with those of a great number of other people. I thank all of you who assisted me, often without your even knowing it.

However, I want to thank in a special way all those who contributed to the realization of this book. The idea of this subject was first suggested to me, with great enthusiasm, by two workshop organizers in German Switzerland (thank you, Stella and David!). When I shared with them what I had learned over many years, from my own diet and from the synthesis I had developed of information on the subject, they eagerly sought to motivate me to write the book as soon as possible. They helped me to realize that this project had already been calling me for some time but I had failed to give it any serious attention.

I want to extend special thanks to my two readers, Micheline St-Jacques and Nathalie Thériault, who were most supportive in the way they executed their task.

A very big thank you to Jean-Pierre Gagnon, managing editor of my publishing house, for his much valued collaboration and his excellent work in the realization of this book.

Untold thanks to my daughter, Monica Shields, CEO of the LISTEN TO YOUR BODY School, for her excellent suggestions following a reading of the first draft. I thank her as well for her remarkable creativity with respect to the design of the cover page and the layout of the book.

Lise Bourbeau

Introduction

Here I am, twenty-seven years after founding my school of life, Listen To Your Body, having the pleasure of conversing with you about everything that we can learn about ourselves by observing our diet. A year before I started my school, in 1981, the idea came to me of noting down everything I ate and drank, because I believed that the cause of my weight gain (20 lbs.) was my diet. Little did I know at that time how that decision would completely transform my life. It was an unforgettable experience, especially the way it triggered my shift from the intellectual to the spiritual world.

Indeed, during the fifteen years that preceded Listen To Your Body, the intellectual aspect was very important to me. As I was working in sales, I was strongly encouraged by my superiors to be interested in positive thinking. At that time, this seemed to be a very important measure of success in the business field. Mental exercises had therefore become the normal approach for me at the first sign of the least little problem I encountered. Although I did obtain positive results from this programming, it did not occur to me that it had to be continually repeated. In fact, I was not getting to the core of the problem. At best, I was managing to control it, by applying these mental practices.

In the months that followed my decision to note down everything I ate and drank each day, I returned to my initial, natural weight, without any control on my part. I discovered that everything I had learned about myself proved to be much more important than solving my weight problem. I had finally become aware of who I was, aware of several of my fears and beliefs; all because I studied the way I ate. Another bonus that came out of this research into my eating patterns was that I noticed, during the months following this work, that numerous physical ailments that had been plaguing me for years disappeared.

That's when I realized that listening to my dietary needs – of a physical nature – would allow me to listen at the same time to my emotional and intellectual needs. I learned that we cannot dissociate these three 'bodies', and that when we work on one of them, it automatically influences the other two. This is why my ailments disappeared. This is how my school of life, LISTEN TO YOUR BODY, began.

Twenty-seven years later, I have finally decided to write this book, in response to an increasing demand by those who have participated in my Listen To Your Body workshops and for the benefit of numerous readers. You will find here everything I learned from my own experience and from that of many others who joined in and shared their results with me.

Just for your information, I want to mention that I use and maintain a familiar style throughout this book as it helps me to communicate the information in a more personal and caring manner.

I want to emphasize that the purpose of this book is not to help you eat in accordance with certain "healthy diet" guidelines. There is no shortage of excellent books on that topic. My goals, rather, are to help you:

> ▶ discover the means of control that you use and how frequently you use them;

► become more aware of your dietary habits;

► make the connection between the way you eat and your emotional, mental and spiritual life;

► discover why it is difficult to listen to your true needs;

► recognize easily the wounds that prevent you from nourishing yourself, physically as well as psychologically;

► develop the ability to listen systematically to your body's needs before you eat;

► love and accept yourself – not only your physical body but, more especially, the person you are, at every moment of everyday.

Happy reading!

Lise Bourbeau

Chapter One

Why is there so much control?

By not using self-control in your life, you give yourself permission to be yourself, whether in the positive or negative sense. You do not burden yourself with judgment or guilt. You accept yourself as you are at every moment of every day.

When you live this way, it is reflected simultaneously in your mental body, your emotional body and your physical body. As the physical body is more visible, tangible and aware, it is the one you can truly rely on when you want to check to find out what is happening in the other two, more subtle, bodies.

The control we all exercise to varying degrees and in different situations starts at the psychological level. Since we cannot dissociate our three bodies, which together form our material envelope, the control – mental or emotional – is immediately reflected in our physical world, including our diet. When you deny yourself chocolate, for example, you might think you are just exercising physical control. But don't be fooled! It is much more than physical. Control is taking place on the other levels at the same time.

The goal then, of the first two chapters of this book, is to help you become aware of the different methods of control you use and how they influence the way you eat.

What is control?

To control yourself or to want to control others means constantly observing and being on guard. It is in fact a desire to dominate, allowing our ego to win at all costs. Indeed it is our ego that fuels all our fears and makes us act and react in accordance with what it believes, because it is sure that way is best for us. Alas, our ego is not aware that every time we are guided by fear, we are no longer being ourselves; we are no longer listening to our true needs. As our ego was generated, exists and survives by virtue of our mental energy, it is made up only of memory, which is to say that it can only live in the past. It is impossible for our ego to know what our deeper self needs at the present moment.

That is why it is so important to become aware of what is directing our life and what is directing the moments when we are in control mode. Furthermore, identifying the means of control that we are using will help us become conscious of one or more of our wounds.

The link between control and our wounds

I have decided to list the means of control that people use, according to the wound that is activated. For those who are not familiar with the five principal wounds of the soul that are taught at the Listen To Your Body School, they are: REJECTION, ABANDONMENT, HUMILIATION, BETRAYAL and INJUSTICE. Each wound is associated with different ways of controlling oneself or controlling others.

Each time you find your life not unfolding in joy, happiness, peace and harmony, it means that every fear, every ailment or illness, every problem you are going through, whether physical, emotional or mental, is an indication that one of your wounds has been activated and that you are in reaction mode. You are no longer yourself; this wound that was touched makes you wear a mask, a different one for each wound. We wear this mask, believing it will protect us from feeling the pain associated with the wound. To learn more about these masks and about the wounds in general, please refer to my book on this subject[1].

I want to remind you that we are all born with most of these five wounds, but in varying degrees. These are the obstacles the soul encounters as it seeks to re-unite itself with the spirit, as it seeks total harmony of being. This is why we are constantly reborn: to become aware of these wounds and enable them to heal, helping ourselves in this way to become our true selves again. These wounds are awakened first of all by our parents – or anyone who played a parental role in our life – from the moment of conception until we reach the age of seven. After that, they are activated by any person who reminds us of any event experienced with either of our parents or with someone who took their place.

In fact, when we react to something because one of our wounds was touched, we are not being ourselves; we are not listening to our true needs, so we go into control mode. A belief associated with the wound that was activated influences us to behave out of one of our fears instead of listening to our needs.

---

[1] *Heal your wounds and find your true self.* Les Editions ETC

I want to remind you that **every fear is a fear for your-self. When you are convinced you are afraid for some-one else, know that the real fear you have is for yourself if, for some reason what you fear for the other person would happen.**

When we believe we are afraid for another person, it is our ego that is playing a trick on us so that we will avoid becoming aware of the true cause of the problem. Let me illustrate with an example. I knew a couple where the wife was continually reminding her husband what he should be eating, when to eat and when to stop. He was diabetic and overweight. She also controlled his medication. One day, my husband and I met them at a restaurant, shortly after they had returned from a weight loss program at a health clinic. It was their first "real" meal in two weeks. When she saw him drinking wine, she started to scowl at him (non-verbal control). Next, she took the bread basket away from him, placing it as far away as possible. She did the same thing with the butter (physical control). She did not dare to express out loud what she was thinking (mental control), but it was easy to sense the anger (emotional level) that she was holding in.

What seemed to bother her most was how much her husband was enjoying everything he ate and drank, and that he was pretending not to notice anything. And the final straw came when for dessert he ordered two scoops of ice cream with whipped cream. At that point, she exploded and started shouting at him in the restaurant that he was a dumb idiot and… I'll spare you the rest. She made a special point of reminding him of the huge amount of money they had just spent at the clinic – all for nothing, she added, still in a rage.

A little later, when I was alone with her, I asked her why she had so much anger. Apparently, it was because she could not manage to control her husband to the same extent that she controlled herself. And finally, she confided to me that she had a great fear of losing her husband if he continued to overeat like this. As I knew she was not telling me about her deeper fear, I persisted with more questions until I learned the exact nature of her own individual fear, if her husband should die.

I learned that her first husband had had very poor eating habits. He was a businessman who was always on the road and he had died of a heart attack. All these years later, she still felt guilty about his death because she was sure that if she had paid more attention to her husband's diet, he would not have died that way. Just the thought of having the death of a second spouse on her conscience made her so anxious that it was turning into an obsession.

Control, fear, belief and wounds

As you may easily conclude, we can observe how in this example control, belief and fear are at work. It tells us that, in this case, two wounds, injustice and betrayal have been activated. The person who has suffered injustice seeks perfection in everything. Consequently, this woman hates herself for not having been the perfect spouse to her first husband and will do anything to make up for that with her second husband. And so she wears the mask of the rigid person. The person who has suffered from betrayal will have difficulty with trust. In this case, she resents the fact that her husband does not trust her, does not appreciate everything she does for him. This woman is wearing the mask of the controller.

She has stopped being herself and has, in particular, stopped listening to her need to enjoy a good meal together with her husband and friends. This woman reacted automatically and went into control mode, indicating that she was wearing the masks associated with her particular wounds.

When a wound is activated

When I talk about an activated wound, I mean that our wounds are always present deep inside us, but that they are not always activated. They become activated when another person awakens them, thus prompting us to react.

It can also happen that one of your wounds becomes activated when there is no one else around. For example, you are home alone and you would love to laze around for a few hours but suddenly a little voice inside your head says you have no right to be lazy and that you should be ashamed of yourself. Even though you are alone, the fear that invades you is occasioned by a belief that you accepted when you were young, generally from one of your parents. This fear of being judged as lazy lives on in you and influences you to be active rather than lazy, out of fear that you will be caught acting lazy or out of fear that someone will judge you as sometimes being lazy. And so, a wound is always activated by your fear of someone, as well as by a belief you hold, to ensure that what you fear doesn't happen.

I even know people who continue to fear their deceased parents. When they dare to behave in a way that goes against what their parents believed, one can immediately discern their fear and guilt when they say, *If my mother could see me now, she would roll over in her grave.* A wound can be activated in any one of three ways, often quite unconsciously: 1) when we are afraid of being hurt by someone else; 2) when we are afraid of hurting someone else; 3) when we hurt ourselves.

We can speak of control not only when we refrain from an action or from being a certain way, but also all the times when we do not manage to control ourselves and have immense feelings of guilt, beating up on ourselves for not having had enough self-control.

Most of the time, we are unaware that a wound has been activated. It is especially our reaction to the situation or person confronting us that can alert us to it. All the methods of controlling indicated in this chapter are a reaction and not a voluntary action. You will see in the next chapter how these reactions influence the way that you eat, which will help you to discover another way of becoming aware that a wound has been activated. What follows are some of the ways we control ourselves, depending on the wound being activated.

The wound of rejection

Let us begin with the wound of REJECTION. How do you control yourself when you are afraid of being rejected, afraid of rejecting someone else or when you reject yourself?

▶   When you rehash endlessly something you are obsessed about having to do or say that raises fear in you, or something that was said concerning you, which touches or awakens your wound;

- ▶ When you suffer from insomnia because your mind is too full of mental activity;

- ▶ When you flee a situation by slipping out quickly from the place where you are or by escaping into faraway thoughts;

- ▶ When you deny a situation, not wanting to see it as it really is. You might be trying to make yourself believe that the person or the situation did not bother you at all, did not affect you, move you or arouse certain emotions in you. This type of control is generally unconscious. It's a good idea to ask those who are close to us to help us recognize those moments when we try to escape through denial;

- ▶ When you deny the veracity or pertinence of a compliment, believing that if that person really knew you, they would never have given it;

- ▶ When you are ashamed of who or what you ARE and desperately do not want anyone to know;

- ▶ When you withdraw and refrain from saying or doing something out of fear that the other will no longer love you or will stop appreciating you.

An important point to remember regarding the wound of REJECTION: it is always activated by fear related to BEING, not DOING or HAVING. For example, if you have to speak or present something to an audience, you might find you over-prepare and then are unable to sleep. Your real fear is not that you will do it wrong, but rather that you will be judged as being a FAILURE if you do not do it perfectly, according to their expectations or that you will not meet your own, mostly unrealistic, expectations.

If you belong to this category of people, it is very likely that you are controlling yourself in what you say and do, mainly because you want to be loved and accepted as you are and do not want to be considered a loser.

The wound of abandonment

Let's move now to the controlling behaviour adopted when you are afraid of being abandoned, afraid of abandoning someone else or when you abandon or give up on yourself.

► When you pretend to be happy and cheerful, in order to please your spouse;

► When you put other people's needs first and convince yourself that this makes you happy;

► When you cry to get what you want or to attract attention;

► When you express your wishes or your unhappiness in a whining tone;

► When you constantly trouble other people in order to get attention;

► When you play the victim, unconsciously attracting problems;

► When you use exaggeration and drama to recount what is happening to you;

► When you take advantage of being sick in order to manipulate the other person, to get them to look after you;

▶ When you do not listen to your own needs, for fear that the other person might think or believe that you are abandoning or ignoring them;

▶ When you start something but then give up, throwing in the towel before you reach your goal, often falsely blaming the person you believe should have supported you;

▶ When you fritter away the time that you are alone, not managing to undertake anything;

▶ When you need to tell someone – on the phone or in person – everything that has happened to you;

▶ When you think you are incapable of facing the imminent death of a loved one;

▶ When you will endure anything out of a fear of being abandoned, usually by a spouse or son or daughter;

▶ When you cannot make the decision to end a relationship out of fear of finding yourself alone again, even when you know it would be better for you;

▶ When you seek help with something, before even trying to see whether you can do it on your own;

▶ When you interrupt another person to talk about your own problems;

▶ When you think that your problems are much bigger than other people's problems.

The wound of humiliation

If you suffer from humiliation, here are the controlling behaviours you most frequently use when you are afraid of humiliating someone else, of being humiliated by someone else or when you humiliate yourself:

- ► When you let another person put you down physically or psychologically without saying anything;

- ► When you consider yourself obliged to help another person with a problem, while forgetting your own needs;

- ► When you prohibit yourself from saying anything whatsoever that is negative about another person;

- ► When you repress your physical desires, with thoughts like *God sees everything* or *God is watching me*;

- ► When you consider yourself unclean, unworthy, dirty;

- ► When you are disgusted with yourself;

- ► When you make others laugh at your expense, thus humiliating yourself;

- ► When you return a compliment to the other person, believing yourself unworthy of receiving it and in particular being convinced that the other person, who is more worthy, deserves it more than you do;

- ► When you do your utmost to be beyond reproach in the eyes of God;

- ► When you think you must alleviate the suffering of others, of humanity;

- ► When you let others go ahead of you, believing they suffer more than you do;

- ► When you do not allow yourself to experience sensual pleasure, for fear you may be seen as a whore;

► When you refuse to offer yourself any physical pleasure, out of fear you may be considered egotistical.

The wound of betrayal

Let us move now to the wound of BETRAYAL, the wound most likely to push us to want to control others. Here are the different methods of control used, when you are afraid of being betrayed by another person or of betraying another person. Do not forget that what you do to others, you do to yourself.

One can suffer from betrayal each time there is a breach of trust, a lie, a promise not kept, an act of cowardice, or a lack of responsibility. Moreover, all the following forms of control are experienced with someone of the opposite sex.

► When you want to have the last word;

► When you lie;

► When you interrupt the other person before they have finished speaking;

► When you jump to conclusions before the other person has finished;

► When you remain bitter and decide not to talk to the other person anymore;

► When you speak loudly and take over completely in a conversation;

► When you don't allow yourself to trust the other person because you are distrustful and you have misgivings about them;

- When you go out of your way to be recognized as a special, strong, capable person;

- When you have expectations without a clear agreement beforehand having been reached;

- When you become impatient because the other person isn't going fast enough;

- When you get angry because things are not going according to your plans;

- When you insist that the other person should agree with you and hold the same opinions as you;

- When you use some form of seduction in order to reach your goals;

- When you blame the other person for your own oversight, error or disloyalty;

- When you watch the other person closely to make sure they carry out their tasks the way you want them to;

- When you ask someone to do something for you and immediately afterwards do not trust them, entertaining doubts about how they are going to carry out your request;

- When you refuse to promise the other person anything;

- When you do not accept responsibility for your actions, wanting the other person to condone your mistake or your oversight;

- When you ridicule the other person as a means of trying to change them;

➤ When you systematically refuse the other person's advice;

➤ When you seek to intimidate the other person;

➤ When you sulk in order to achieve your goal and get your way;

➤ When you shout at or threaten the other person;

➤ When you try to impose your way of doing things;

➤ When you make a decision for the other person without consulting them.

The wound of injustice

I end with the wound of injustice, which is experienced by those who are too perfectionist and who easily accuse themselves. They use the following means of control with themselves and with people of the same sex. Below are the aspects of your behaviour that show up when you're afraid that someone will treat you unjustly or you're afraid of treating yourself or someone else unjustly or in a less than perfect manner:

➤ When you do not respect your limits and you ask too much of yourself;

➤ When you pretend you are doing fine even when you are not;

➤ When you justify your actions by distorting reality;

➤ When you refuse to ask for help, believing that you can do it better yourself;

➤ When you hold back from showing your feelings;

► When you hold back your tears or cry only in private;

► When you judge the other person as being over-sensitive;

► When you refuse to allow yourself to take medication or consult a doctor;

► When you revise what you have just done, several times;

► When you start the same task over numerous times;

► When you interrupt the other person, judging their remarks to be untrue or unfair;

► When you try to get others to tell you that what you have just accomplished is perfect;

► When you want a quick, immediate solution to a problem before you have taken the time to be with it or figure out the cause;

► When you judge or accuse the other person of having behaved badly or wrongly;

► When you want to be considered right because you are sure you have the right answer;

► When you experience anger because you feel a situation cannot be justified;

► When you criticize yourself severely, thinking it will help you to improve;

► When you engage in self-destructive behaviour or under-estimate yourself whenever you achieve success;

► When you refuse to receive anything whatsoever from another person, for fear of becoming indebted toward them;

- ▶ When you say yes when you want to say no, out of fear of being unfair or insensitive;

- ▶ When you fail to do yourself a favour because you think you don't deserve it;

- ▶ When you force yourself to smile or laugh;

- ▶ When you are a workaholic out of fear that someone will think you are lazy;

- ▶ When you rationalize with yourself that you want something while you really want something else, instead of listening to your heart;

- ▶ When you criticize the other person for not pulling up their socks;

- ▶ When you fail to show your anger;

- ▶ When you don't allow yourself to be happy, if there is someone close to you who is not happy.

It is possibly more difficult to recognize the controlling behaviours of the last two wounds because the controlling person and the rigid person have a larger ego. These are two strong wounds which trigger faster and more intense reactions. The stronger our ego, the more it is able to make us believe what it wants, for example that we are right and that the other person is wrong.

Becoming conscious of the extent of our control

I strongly suggest you take the time to read over these methods of control a few times, so that it will be easier to see how they connect with the information in Chapter Two. Here is the way to proceed. Write down the control methods that you use, with whom (child, spouse, family, friends, coworkers) and in what circumstances. To facilitate this exercise, here are several areas where control is used:

- ➢ Physical appearance;
- ➢ Manner of dress;
- ➢ Use of money or budgeting;
- ➢ Household chores and duties at work;
- ➢ Going out, recreation, vacation;
- ➢ Choice of friends;
- ➢ Studies;
- ➢ Choice of professional life;
- ➢ Signs of attention and affection;
- ➢ Sexuality;
- ➢ Attitude, behaviour;
- ➢ Religion, spiritual development.

There is nothing wrong with asking those close to you what control mechanisms they see you using. However, it does take a certain amount of humility. But if you are reading this book, I suspect you want to challenge yourself to improve your quality of life.

Additionally, if you want to go a step further, take the time to check, in each situation, what kinds of accusations or judgments you make toward others and toward yourself. Afterwards, you may try and define some of the fears you have for yourself. I will come back to this type of analysis in the final chapter.

You will see just how useful it can be for you to know what type of control you are seeking to exercise in your life, as reflected in either your loss of control or your efforts to control, with respect to food. Let's take a look now at the link between the way you eat and any one of your wounds that becomes activated.

Chapter Two

The link between control and eating

I mentioned in the preceding chapter that our wounds are awakened during the first seven years of life – starting from the moment we are born – by our parents and all those who filled a parental role toward us during that time. Thereafter, each time a wound is activated by anyone at all, it is simply a repetition of something that has already happened but of which we are unaware.

Let us take the example of a little girl who felt rejected from the moment she was born because her mother was disappointed at not having had a boy. Her wound of rejection was awakened at the moment she was born or, more likely, while still in the fetal state. Consequently, regardless of what her mother said or did, it is very probable that the little girl, the adolescent and, later, the young woman, always misinterpreted her mother's behaviour. In fact, it is very important to remember that what causes our suffering is not what another person does, but rather our reaction, as influenced by one of our wounds.

This can explain why it is not uncommon for two children who have different wounds to have a very different experience of a parent's behaviour toward them, even when the parent acts the same way toward each child.

The influence of the mother's behaviour

When it comes to the question of diet, it is the influence of the mother (or of whoever played the role of mother during the first seven years of life) that is felt the most. Why? Because the mother symbolizes mother Earth and the father symbolizes our father, the Sun. The Earth – which we also call All-Nourishing Mother – nourishes us with her abundant garden. She provides us with our basic sustenance. It is also in the nature of things for the mother to have the role of nourishing our inner life, that is, of helping us to feel well. As for the father, his role is to help us apply our energy toward being creative, taking action and obtaining material security.

As soon as it is born, the baby needs the mother's milk. It is the most natural thing in the world – and this is true for all animals – to see a baby wanting to suckle immediately after it is born. It seeks its mother's breast. This is why it is so important for the mother to offer her breast to her infant. Even if she cannot do it for long, it is crucial in the first few weeks, as part of the start and preparation of this child's entire life, according to the natural order of things.

When a mother cannot breastfeed her child, or refuses to do so, the child's experience of this, in the case of a female child, activates her wound of rejection in a major way. In the case of a male child, it is the wound of abandonment that is activated by this experience. In my book about wounds, I explain clearly why each wound is awakened by a specific parent.

I want to remind you that when a child experiences a certain wound with a parent, the parent experiences the same wound himself or herself even though most of the time, they will not be aware of it. Our children have the gift of bringing to the surface issues in us that we have not yet resolved with our own parents. Sometimes a baby is unable to digest its mother's milk or refuses to suckle. This often represents the wound of rejection or abandonment being activated in the mother.

In the example of a mother who cannot breastfeed her daughter, if the daughter feels rejected, the mother's wound of rejection is also activated. The mother, consciously or not, berates herself for not being able to breastfeed her baby. It is very possible that she is afraid she will hurt her baby and that her baby will not love her. By searching a little deeper within herself, she will undoubtedly discover that she experienced the same thing with her own mother. As soon as any such emotion surfaces, a wound is activated.

At the same time, the baby who refuses to accept its mother's nourishment has a greater risk of suffering from anorexia later on. I will return to this point in a later chapter.

So, the behaviour and inner attitude of the mom, with respect to food, influences the child a lot. Generally, this behaviour will be unconscious on the mom's part because she doesn't realize that the reason she is behaving this way with her child is that she needs to engage in this type of behaviour in order to become aware of her own wounds. Indeed, it is not just by chance that parents act a certain way with their children. Everything is already written into each family's life plan. Parents act out of their own woundedness in the way they relate to their children's wounds.

This makes it possible for all family members to engage in mutually assisting one another to become more aware and eventually to succeed in healing their wounds.

It has been observed that when a baby cries and parents don't quite know what to do or are upset by it, the mother will decide to give the baby, even in early infancy, something sweet in its mouth. I say "the mother" because usually she's the one who dictates how the child should be fed. Of course there are exceptions to every rule, but for the purposes of this book, I will stick to the general rule of what happens in the majority of cases.

Not so long ago, we would still be giving a child a pacifier that had been dipped in sugar or honey, or a bottle of juice without really knowing if it was what the baby needed. Over time, it became a habit and we continued to do this. If a child cried or got hurt, was rambunctious or bored, or was disturbing others, we gave them something sweet to eat or drink. While we are still very young, we learn to respond to our slightest emotional upsets by filling ourselves with anything at all to eat or drink except what we may actually need. The vast majority of people have thus learned to get the attention and comfort they seek by rewarding themselves with something they can pop into their mouth.

This is why each time one of your wounds is activated, it is hard for you to know if you really are hungry and, *if* you are, to know what your body really needs. Depending on which wound is activated, you will tend to eat or drink in a different way.

The wound of rejection
and the way you eat

(Mask: withdrawer)

When it is the wound of rejection that you are dealing with and that is influencing you to control yourself, it is more likely that you will have a diminished appetite. You no longer feel anything; you don't even feel that your body needs food. And if you do eat, you will be particularly inclined to take small portions. You will just use the tip of your fork, being more or less unaware of what is on your plate and not really tasting what you eat. The mask of the withdrawer that appears with this wound means you are no longer really present to what is taking place in the physical world.

As a result, while being more interested in the mental aspect of the world than things relating to the physical world, you are unable to really enjoy your food. The most common food used for escape is sugar, sugar in all its forms, when drugs or alcohol are not an option. Furthermore, I have noticed in persons wearing the mask of the withdrawer that sugar very often produces effects similar to those of alcohol.

Eating a large amount of sugar sets off a vicious cycle in your body and can furthermore be quite harmful. Your body, principally your suprarenal glands, will have to work very hard in order to absorb and eliminate this sugar; your body will become weakened and tired. When you feel lacking in energy, you will reach for something containing sugar again in the hope of recovering this lost energy. But this is the wrong way, because the renewed energy will not last long and therefore you will have to repeat the cycle over and over.

The withdrawer will also prefer very spicy foods. It is another way of tasting something in order to obtain certain sensations. Unable to taste the real flavour of each food, this person reasons that at least they will taste the spices. This can explain why some people can eat very spicy food without reacting to it.

The wound of abandonment
and the way you eat

(Mask: dependent)

When it is the wound of abandonment that you are dealing with and that is influencing you to be controlling, it is the opposite that takes place. You seek love outside yourself, in the form of attention, affection and support. You don't know how to obtain it and so you compensate for it in your diet. Not receiving from others what you want from them, you try to satisfy your need in the form of food. This has you able to eat non-stop –believing that you can fill the inner emptiness you are experiencing. You eat a lot, not because it tastes good or because your body needs it but rather to give yourself the impression of getting what you are lacking. Despite constantly stuffing yourself, you nevertheless continue to feel like your stomach is empty. It feels like a bottomless pit. What you do not realize is that the emptiness is rather in your heart. As food cannot replace the lack in your affective life, you feel you never have enough and you don't know when to stop. It is your heart that needs to be filled, with a good dose of self-love.

I have also noticed that when someone is wearing their dependency mask and is taking their meal in good company, they will often eat very slowly to make the pleasure last longer. It is their way of controlling the amount of attention they need. They are also more drawn to soft foods, which don't require a great deal of chewing.

The wound of humiliation and the way you eat

(Mask: masochist)

When you suffer from the wound of humiliation, you use control in order not to enjoy your senses because you believe that it is undignified to be a sensual person. In front of others, you will often refrain from eating what you like most; you will force yourself to choose what you think is appropriate for a good person. However, there comes a time when the masochist can no longer restrain themselves, their senses having, in a way, been held hostage. They lose their control over food and eat exaggerated quantities, because it is JUST SO GOOD. Furthermore, you sense the pleasure you will derive from eating food just by seeing it. If you see yourself as this kind of person, it will certainly be very difficult for you to pass by a tray of snacks without having something. When you know there are sweets or other foods you like at home, it must be very hard for you to resist them. You know you are not hungry but you cannot help yourself.

The masochist enjoys food physically, but takes little pleasure from it psychologically. The greater their physical enjoyment, the greater their guilt in letting themselves go, in whatever area. They often eat to fill up rather than because they are in tune with their body. They believe that if they feel hungry, they will become aware of their body, which to them is somehow unspiritual.

Once they have started eating, they find plenty of reasons to continue. *Since I've already gone overboard and have surely gained a pound or two already, I might as well keep going,* they think. All this to prove to themselves that they are unworthy, shameful, piggish or too fond of food. The masochistic tendency shows up in the form of the suffering and punishment they impose on themselves. They suffer when they are hungry and they suffer when they have eaten too much.

This type of person is especially attracted by fatty foods like butter, cream, rich sauces, etc. They might continue this way until they become disgusted with what they are eating, just as much as they are disgusted with themselves.

The wound of betrayal
and the way you eat

(Mask: controller)

With the wound of betrayal, since you want to have control over what's going on around you and you have trouble trusting others, you duplicate the same pattern in your own diet. The expression "to take it with a grain of salt" applies very well to the controller.

You know this is your mask if you make sure to add salt or pepper, spices or sugar, etc. whenever someone else has prepared the meal. How many times have I not seen people add a liberal dose of salt and pepper to their meal before they have even tasted it!

I remember one day noticing a couple seated at the table next to mine in a restaurant. The man received his plate and as he continued talking to his companion, he took the salt shaker and sprinkled salt all over the food on his plate. Being curious, I could not help but count the number of times he repeated this gesture. Eighteen times!!! I observed him closely, telling myself that he had surely been unaware of what he had done and would be unable to swallow any of his food. But no, he ate it all. However, he ate like the true controller, never taking the time to chew properly or to taste the food, as he ate far too quickly.

You know that this wound has been activated if you are doing numerous other things while you are eating, like reading, discussing business or lecturing your children or your spouse during a family meal, watching TV, etc. This is why you are not really paying attention to what you are putting in your mouth and there is a great likelihood you are eating more than necessary, mainly because you are ingesting everything so rapidly. Some even swallow huge portions without chewing them first. This way, it is impossible for the stomach to pick up the brain's message telling it that it has had enough.

Controllers also bite into their food. They want so much to control others that when they experience anger in the face of their expectations not being met, they try to assuage their hunger by biting. This is often the reason for eating meat, not because their body needs it but because of the need to bite.

They can appear to be people who really enjoy their food, because they are avid eaters and love tasting everything. However, if they are in control mode, that is, in their wound, the reality is different. Convinced of their own so-called well-being, they may often say *Is that ever good*. But they eat very quickly without really tasting.

The wound of injustice
and the way you eat

(Mask: rigid)

If you are operating out of your wound of injustice, you will deal with your food the same way you deal with life. You will try to control yourself as much as possible. Only those who suffer from this wound succeed in following a draconian diet and controlling themselves to achieve their ideal weight or the waist they consider acceptable.

When your rigid persona gets into gear, you are able to control the quantity and selection of foods you take in. It is very possible, moreover, that you judge the behaviour of those who "let themselves go" so harshly that you regularly declare things like *I NEVER take sugar or dessert. I NO LONGER drink alcohol. I ONLY eat health foods. I NEVER snack between meals.* You glory so much in your capacity to control yourself that you do not notice that you are making statements that do not correspond to reality at all. People who wear the rigid mask like to use superlatives like *always, never, extraordinary, incredible*, etc.

I have a friend who, whenever she eats at my home, always says the same thing when it comes time for dessert: I am so proud of myself; I have stopped taking dessert for some time now. But today, I'll make an exception. You're such a great cook and this dessert looks so delicious that I'm going to let myself be tempted. I will refrain here from telling you how much dessert she consumes. I am convinced that she is unaware of this "maneuver" that she has been engaging in for several years and is even less aware of how much dessert she eats.

Earlier, I spoke of the masochist who was eating too much, and feeling guilty all the while. The rigid person feels very guilty too but as he or she excels in self-control, rationalizing is easy to do. They can make themselves believe that it's not serious since it's only this once. That way, they try to hide their guilt feelings from themselves. This attitude brings on physical problems that can be sudden and very painful, which appear in order to draw the person's attention to all the guilt they are hiding. Moreover, they have real trouble finding the cause of their problems, as they are not conscious of what it is they feel guilty about. The various pains brought on by their behaviour are in fact their unconscious attempt to punish themselves.

If the rigid person ever ends up losing control with respect to food or drink, having exceeded their limit in other areas, they will do their utmost to deal with the situation alone and not dare to speak about it. When they lose their control in front of others, their sense of guilt is greatly increased and they promise themselves never to slide again.

The more the rigid person is demanding toward themselves and the more they do not allow themselves to feel, the more inclined they will also be to add spices to their food. However, in contrast to the controlling person, they taste their food first, as everything must be perfect and to their taste. Only then do they add the spices they think they need at that particular time.

The rigid person also likes crunchy foods like chips and will prefer fresh fruits and vegetables that are raw and hard.

If you see yourself in this wound, it is very possible that you are the kind of person who reads all the food labels carefully, checking the ingredients and quantities. Are you really doing this because you love yourself – because you refuse to eat chemical additives, for example? Or is it because you are afraid you might find fattening ingredients?

I have often observed rigid people who, when they lose control, eat huge quantities of non-fattening foods; they tell themselves that's not so bad. Nevertheless, the body is not any happier, because it has to figure out how to digest, absorb, and eliminate or store this surplus somewhere in the organism. The same is true for sugar, even if it is natural the absorption of a large quantity of sugar will inevitably be damaging to the body.

You might also be upset when people around you eat large quantities. As you permit yourself this luxury only rarely, it will be hard for you to accept someone else allowing themselves what you perceive as an indulgence. To be entitled to eat as much as you want, especially of the foods you really like, you believe it must be deserved. If it is not deserved, you impose restrictions on yourself.

So often, I have seen people eating with enjoyment, love and appetite when, suddenly for no apparent reason, they push their plate away, saying *That's enough. I have to stop now.* You can even note a certain stiffness in their manner. They have donned their rigid mask and decided it is time to control themselves.

44

I want to remind you that all these controls and losses of control related to the five wounds are a reflection of another type of control, taking place in your psychological life. The physical is always a reflection of what is going on beyond the body's envelope. This is why it is useless to apply physical control, because the cause of your controlling behaviour can be found only beyond the physical and will continue to persist. It is as if you are trying to hide an infected wound with a band-aid without caring for it properly, in the hope that if you don't see it, it will go away. Of course, it is just the opposite because now the wound will actually get worse.

This applies to all physical problems, which, according to medical knowledge, are caused by poorly managed diets that fail to respect the body's needs. Liver attacks, indigestion, heartburn, hypoglycemia, diabetes, intestinal problems, etc. are good examples of ailments or conditions that will often require a change in dietary habits.

These physical problems are expressions of your deeper self, which is trying to draw attention to inner attitudes you have that are no longer beneficial to you. The Divine in you is trying to tell you, through these ailments that it is high time for you to learn to love yourself more. Since I have written an entire book[2] covering some five hundred ailments and illnesses, I will not be listing them in the present work.

---

[2] *Your body's telling you : Love yourself!*, Lise Bourbeau, Editions ETC, 2001

Choosing your foods

To conclude this chapter, here is a summary of the meaning of the various food choices and behaviours that are the most common. Your choices and behaviours are another way of becoming aware of your wounds. In the fourth chapter, you will find a quick and simple method to help you get to know yourself better, based on your dietary habits. The statements that follow refer not only to the foods you eat but also to everything you drink, with the exception of water.

For each of the foods mentioned below, a number of explanations are given. It may be that only one or perhaps several will apply to you.

Salty foods or too much salt: voicing your opinion about what others say or do. Finding it hard not to have the last word. Needing to be right. Wanting everything to go according to your wishes. Afraid of being controlled. Putting unnecessary pressure on yourself, given that it is impossible to control everything. Having trouble expressing yourself when you would like to have the last word.

How do you know if you are consuming too much salt? There is a good chance that you are part of the majority of people who consume too much salt. The daily minimum requirement is half a gram. The ideal amount is one and a half grams. In North America, the average amount of sodium consumed daily is seven grams, that is, more than four times the ideal amount recommended. Large amounts of salt are used as a preservative in the ready-made and processed foods available at the supermarket. Health professionals tell us this is one of the main reasons why nine out of ten Canadians suffer from high blood pressure. It is not actually the salt that causes the high blood pressure, but the emotions you have that make you absorb too much salt.

Sweets or sugar: lack of sweetness in your life. Being too demanding of yourself, asking too much of yourself. Trouble complimenting yourself or recognizing your true worth. Believing you are entitled to a reward only when you have accomplished something extraordinary. Afraid of being egotistical. Not being in contact with all that you receive, believing that you are lacking, meaning that you are more in touch with what you do not receive compared to your expectations.

How do you know if you are consuming too much sugar? The various results of research on this topic show differing conclusions. On the other hand, I have often heard that the quantity of sugar present in three fresh fruits is more than sufficient to meet your daily requirement. Therefore, anything over that would represent indulgence.

Spicy foods or spices: a lack of spice in your life, which means an inability to sense beauty, the marvelousness of what surrounds you and especially the greatness of your inner self. An absence of passion, either in your love life, your career or your life in general. Allowing the mental and analytical to take up all the space rather than really feeling what is going on in you and being passionate about life. Fear of feeling. Not being sufficiently in touch with and grateful for the small moments of excitement in your life.

Foods that are rich in fat: disgust with yourself, whether physically or psychologically. Guilt. Wanting to punish yourself to the point of stuffing your body with the very foods that are the hardest for it to digest, absorb and eliminate. Believing that you deserve to be punished if you look after yourself before you look after others.

Crunchy or crusty foods: being too strict and demanding with yourself. Believing that your life has to be tough and difficult. Giving yourself a lot of hassle, worrying for nothing, making your life complicated when it doesn't need to be. Believing you must earn your heavenly reward by the sweat of your brow. Beating up on yourself when you see yourself as a spineless or lazy person. Quick to criticize others, showing impatience and intolerance toward them.

Soft foods: lacking the strength and perseverance to build the life you want. Counting on others for your happiness. Believing you can't achieve anything by yourself. Criticizing yourself for wanting a happy, easy life, wanting to take it easy. Believing that when you act like a strong person, people won't bother with you anymore.

Caffeine: showing a lack of stimulation in your life, that is, having very few goals that motivate you, that make you keen to get up in the morning. You get involved in other people's goals and projects rather than your own.

A lot of bread: Never having your fill of bread – bread being the basic human nourishment – means you believe you are not being sufficiently nourished by those close to you. You are dependent, either on their presence, their attention, their compliments, their gratitude or their opinion, and this constitutes a kind of support system for you.

～

I want to clarify that what I have described above is not meant to become or degenerate into an obsession. All these descriptions are of moments when you realize you have

48

gone beyond what is normal. For example, your appetite for spaghetti (a soft food) is not an indication that you rely on others to create your happiness for you. On the other hand, if you crave pasta several times a week, the definition given above probably does apply to you.

The same is true for all the examples given. If you drink one or two coffees a day, that is very different from having several and not even knowing how many cups you have consumed.

Various behaviours

For each of the behaviours mentioned below, a number of explanations are given. It may be that only one or perhaps several will apply to you.

Eating or drinking very slowly: wanting to make the enjoyment last longer, seeking attention, seeking someone's company. Fear of solitude.

Eating or drinking very quickly: not being present to your meal, because you are trying to control something or someone else. Wanting to control time. Being afraid others will think you are slow, irresponsible and/or untrustworthy. Wanting to win, gain the upper hand over someone else. Fear of not being good enough.

Eating or drinking very little: believing you do not deserve to be nourished by your mother or by whatever relates to maternal love. Not being in touch with our own needs. Fear of being loved becomes stronger than the desire to be loved. Not eating or drinking enough is often an indication that there is a "too much" in another area where you do not accept yourself. It may also mean that you are able to manage this area of excess, but without realizing it.

Eating or drinking too much: filling up until you feel sick, not being in touch with your limits. Wanting to take on or do too much for others. Seeing that your family members are pampered, all to the detriment of your own needs. Fear of not being loved. Punishing yourself, suffering from having overeaten. Eating or drinking too much is often an indication that there is a lack in another area where you do not accept yourself. It may also be a matter of being "fed up" without realizing it.

Biting into your food: wishing to "bite" someone. Controlling your anger. Building up expectations without anyone having promised anything – even implicitly. Wanting everything to go your way. Afraid of being gentle and vulnerable, and criticizing yourself for it when you are.

To swallow directly without tasting: wishing someone would get out of your life. Having resentment, holding a grudge. Refusing to see and recognize the other person's good side. Rejecting the other person's way of being. Fear of being vulnerable. The phenomenon of not tasting anything also shows that this person has trouble tasting the pleasures of life, hating themselves when taking the liberty of doing so.

Chapter Three

Do you know your body's needs?

In order to get to know yourself through your food intake, the first thing to find out is whether you listen properly to your body's physical needs. When you are conscious of listening to your body, it means that you are listening just as much to your emotional and mental bodies and their needs. If you are not listening to your physical body, you will consequently learn that the same is true for the other "bodies".

Our three bodies, which constitute our material envelope and allow us to live on this planet, cannot be dissociated from one another. Everything that happens in one body automatically affects the other two. It is therefore wiser to be alert to what you experience in your physical body, as it is more concrete than the other two.

That is why I am reminding you of what it means to "listen to the needs of your physical body". Although most of us learned these things in earliest childhood, it is important to call them to mind again. Our physical body needs:

- ◆ to breathe (air);
- ◆ to drink (water);
- ◆ to eat (food/nourishment);
- ◆ to move (physical exercise);

♦   to rest and to sleep.

In this chapter, I'll be dwelling especially on the need to eat – we will look at the other needs in Chapter Six. If you are like me, when we were young and heard people talk about eating what was good for you, we understood: "only eat boring food" or "deny yourself anything delicious" or "if it's good for your health, it's bound to taste awful" or possibly, "be careful about everything you eat" (which represents a lot of work). And what about you? What does your brain register, when you hear that it's important to listen to the dietary needs of your physical body?

My purpose in reviewing these needs is not to get you to take "control". Far from it. In fact I know today that this is hardly the solution. That is why I discourage any form of control, whether on the physical or the emotional and mental levels. My intention is above all to help you realize that your body – which is your vehicle in this life – is like any other type of "carriage": If it is not maintained and given adequate attention and care, it will not last as long and will not be able to function at full capacity.

Let me remind you the main reasons why we need to eat:

▶   To ensure our physical and psychic growth and development

▶   To maintain a healthy body

▶   To preserve the body's natural immunity

▶   To ensure continuation of the species.

So, we do not eat in the first instance for the pleasure of tasting or to satisfy our hunger. Those two reasons should be secondary in people's minds. That is the main reason why we need to be cautious about the food choices we make and the quality of what we ingest.

The six essential nutrients

Your body needs six nutrients to function properly. It will let you know which one it needs when you feel hungry or thirsty. It may need water, protein, lipids (fat), carbohydrates (sugar), vitamins or minerals.

When you ingest any other element, you give your body a big chore to do, depleting some of its energy, in contrast to the desired goal of good nutrition, which is to help your body build energy. It indicates that you are not listening to your needs, in general. For example, refined sugars, white starch, non-essential fats, alcohol, tobacco, caffeine and any chemicals (including medications) are all ingredients that require a lot of work on the part of your body's digestive, absorptive and eliminative functions.

You will learn, in this book, what motivates you to nourish your body one way rather than another. I have yet to meet a person who ALWAYS listens to their body's needs. What is reassuring is that our body is extraordinarily strong and flexible and knows through its innate intelligence, that the natural state of the human is to live in harmony. To achieve this harmony, we need to learn to love ourselves more, before we can succeed in listening to our real needs, on all levels.

I have no intention whatsoever of making you feel guilty when you notice that you do not listen to your needs. This new consciousness is to be used ONLY for the purpose of helping you get to know yourself.

With respect to the six essential nutrients, it is of course important to remember that the more natural the ingredients are, the happier your body will be by virtue of its digestive system not having to work as hard.

Water. After air, this is our body's greatest need, as water constitutes about 65% of our body. Water is necessary for the blood and the tissues, as well as to transport nutrients, eliminate waste and help the body regulate its temperature.

When you are thirsty, all your body needs is pure water. If you take a drink of pure water, rather than a drink of water filled with chemicals, it makes a significant difference. To see the proof, place a glass of pure water at room temperature beside a glass of impure water – for example, water that has been treated with chlorine – for twenty-four hours. Then, taste the water from each glass. This experiment will tell you what it means to drink pure water.

Moreover, it is good to remember that your body regularly needs at least two liters of water per day, in order to replace what you lose through your urine, from perspiring, and through the pores of your skin. Unfortunately, you cannot include in those two liters any water or other liquid that has been converted into a drink of coffee or tea or any other drink. As soon as water loses the key quality of being absolutely pure, that is, of being only H_2O and nothing else, it means the liquid must be filtered by the digestive system. Pure water, on the other hand, is absorbed by the body as it is.

Each of us is capable of adopting new habits. Have you noticed the ease with which a person who has decided to take up smoking always remembers their pack of cigarettes? As you can see, all it takes is a decision. So, how about deciding to always remember your personal water bottle? For the first few weeks, you might need to put some reminder notes in an obvious spot so that you think of it. But I can assure you that this good habit can only benefit you.

You also need to remember that as soon as your body is thirsty, any other drink you take will not really be able to quench that thirst. On the contrary, it will only make it worse! Did you know, for instance, that a bottle of cola contains the equivalent of eight teaspoons of sugar? And that for every cup of coffee you drink, your body eliminates twice that amount of water? What this means is that if your body has to handle four cups of coffee a day, it will need four additional glasses of water – in addition to the two liters recommended daily. Note that beer has the same effect as coffee in this regard.

Let us now touch on the other five nutrients briefly, for as you know, the main purpose of this book is not to teach you healthy eating habits. It is designed to help you get to know yourself through the way you eat rather than to help you have control.

Protein. Protein is necessary for the building, maintenance and repair of our cells. Protein fosters growth, for example, the growth of hair, nails, etc.

If you ingest natural protein, as found in legumes, nuts, grains and cereals, it is much easier for your body to use than animal protein. If you nourish your body with animal protein that comes from a contented animal, that is, one that is raised out in nature, rather than in an "animal factory", this also makes a difference.

Lipids. Their most important role, among others, is to bring to the body a concentrated source of energy and to maintain an energy reserve in the adipose tissues. The lipids are of great importance for a healthy skin.

The body, for its part, needs especially unsaturated fats that are plant-based. Saturated fats, of animal origin, are not essential fatty acids. While our body needs essential fatty acids, it is unable to produce them.

Carbohydrates. We all need carbs, our principal source of energy. Likewise, the brain is nourished only by carbohydrates. They exist in the form of sugar or starch. However, it is the natural sugars and the unbleached starches that we should look for.

The carbs the body needs most must come from natural sugars like those contained in fruits. As it takes Vitamin B to transform carbohydrates into energy, what happens when we ingest refined sugars – which don't contain any Vitamin B – is that instead of providing our body with the necessary energy, we are using it up in order to eliminate these useless carbohydrates. And when they are not eliminated, they are stored in the body.

A natural sugar that is easy to absorb and has a very low glycemic index is agave nectar.

❧

You can easily obtain information about the six essential nutrients from other books or any of several Web sites.

This would allow you to check to what extent you are demanding a lot of extra work and effort from your body. Already you can see that if you are making it difficult for your body to digest, absorb and eliminate what you drink and eat, it means you are doing the same thing in your day-to-day life: you are asking too much of yourself, you still do not love yourself enough to make your life easier. In a later chapter, we will look at the more precise significance of various foods.

Chewing

Another factor to be taken into account is chewing. The more you chew, the more you activate the salivary glands, which secrete saliva. This has several functions:

♦   it cleans the mouth;

♦   it dissolves the chemical elements in the food so that the taste can be perceived, thus allowing the pleasure of tasting to be prolonged;

♦   it moistens the food, aiding the process of compacting it into a ball of food (bolus);

♦   it produces enzymes that break down fats in order to start the process of digestion and make the stomach's work easier;

♦   it regulates the pH in the mouth, preventing acid from attacking the teeth thus preserving them.

When you swallow your food as it is, you are skipping this pre-digestion stage and creating problems for the main digestion stage. As a result, you are denying yourself several of the good nutrients that food provides for a human being. Don't you think it is unfortunate if you are selecting good foods that are as natural as possible, yet not benefitting from them as fully as possible?

Another benefit of chewing well is that it helps bring out the nutrients in all the foods we eat – especially the most natural foods –, not only for our physical body, but also for our emotional and mental "bodies". Proper chewing lets us take optimal advantage of all the benefits food offers. Additionally, chewing well on both sides of your mouth allows you to get the real taste of what you are eating, connecting with both the feminine and masculine principles within you. If when you ingest food, you are aware that your three "bodies" (physical, emotional and mental) are being energized and that you are nourishing your masculine and feminine aspects as well, it is highly likely that you will become more attentive to what you choose to eat and will be able to listen more carefully to your body's dietary needs. You will also start to notice that foods become a lot tastier.

Eating slowly and tasting

Chewing properly also aids in stretching out the amount of time it takes to satisfy your appetite. I am not saying this casually it is important that you really take your time when you eat. Furthermore, that doesn't necessarily mean you have to take long breaks between mouthfuls. As far as I am concerned, the best way I have discovered to check whether I am eating slowly or not is to see whether I really taste what I ingest. People like me, who generally do things very rapidly, cannot eat as slowly as people who are slower by nature. I have often heard the suggestion to put down your knife and fork between mouthfuls. The important thing, in

any event, is to find the method that produces the best result for you.

For my part, when I take the time to chew on both sides
of my mouth and I truly taste my food and use my taste
buds, I feel that my body is satisfied. Why is it important to
taste? So that you know in time when your hunger has been
satisfied. Generally speaking, **it is much harder for most
of us to know when we are no longer hungry than it is to
know when we are hungry**. Have you noticed what happens when you have a bad cold and a stuffed-up nose? It is
almost impossible to really taste and savour what you are
eating. Consequently you have the impression you have not
eaten your fill and you keep feeling dissatisfied and hungry
even when you just finished a meal a half hour earlier.

Eating slowly, by the way, has nothing to do with how
long you take to finish your meal. Some people talk incessantly while eating, others answer the phone, get up several
times to attend to other concerns, read a magazine or a
book they find so absorbing they forget to eat. If any of
these scenarios fit you, you must surely have noticed that
you really do not taste (or hardly taste) your food! Although the meal may have required a lot of preparation
time, the mouthfuls could be swallowed quickly.

Let me remind you that not tasting your food when you
eat is an indication that you are having difficulty tasting the
pleasures of life.

Giving your body
what it needs

It may be that you eat exclusively nourishing good food, but do you give your body what it needs when it needs it?

To find out, all you have to do is take a few seconds before you eat or drink and ask yourself, *DO I REALLY NEED THIS RIGHT NOW?* The first few times, it is almost certain that you won't quite know how to answer the question. We are so skilled at making ourselves believe all sorts of things that it is very easy to say, *Yes, yes, I really feel like having this cake right now.*

Let's take a few seconds to look at the difference between a need and a desire. We much more frequently desire something that does not actually meet our body's needs than we seek what truly does meet its needs. Suppose you are at home and you know there are some delicious little chocolates in a drawer. Just thinking about these chocolates makes your mouth water. It is possible you need them. In order to be sure, ask yourself the following question: *If there wasn't any in the drawer, would I have thought about chocolate?* If you spontaneously answer *YES*, and you are even prepared to go out and get some anywhere you can, it is very likely that you really do need them.

Another way to know if this desire corresponds to a need is to wait at least a half hour and if, at the end of that period of time, you have forgotten that you wanted them, it was just a passing whim. But if the thought persists, it indicates a genuine need.

However, is this need physical or psychological? To know this, ask yourself first of all if you are really hungry.

60

Because wanting to eat and being hungry are two different things. If you left the table barely an hour ago, you cannot really be hungry. It's just a craving for chocolate that you have and most likely this "gourmandise" is trying to meet a psychological need, like the need for company, reward, reassurance, acknowledgment or recognition. If this is the case, eat the chocolate, even if your physical body doesn't really need it. At the very least, you can be grateful that you became aware of your psychological need at that moment. You will realize that when you ingest food or liquid, while being aware that it is very likely something else that you really need, you will be able to stop eating it sooner and more easily. Gradually, you will find another way to satisfy that need.

When you experience hunger, your body is attracting your attention in its way, by creating various noises and sensations. By becoming more alert, you will soon recognize what your personal signals are that let you detect real hunger. These signals vary from one person to another. There is no need to worry about learning to recognize them easily; your body is so perfect that it knows exactly when it is hungry and what it needs. If you believe or think you might be hungry, it is a sign that you are not really famished. It's a bit like asking someone whether they have a back ache and they answer *I think it hurts*. From such a response, you can logically deduce they do not really have a sore back.

Do you trust your body when it lets you know it needs for you to pass water or have a bowel movement? Do you need to remind your body when to perspire or how to heal a wound? This applies to all bodily functions. In fact, it is the most sophisticated machine in the world and is, moreover, equipped with its own intelligence. You don't have to decide for your body the times when it is hungry.

When you are sure you are hungry and to ensure you give your body what it needs, the following questions will prove to be very useful:

► *What are my taste buds telling me?*

► *Eat something warm? Something cold?*

► *Something hard? Something soft?*

► *Something sweet? Not sweet?*

With a little practice, you will be pleasantly surprised to note how quickly these questions can be asked and answered. You might, for example, hear the message: something warm, soft and not sweet. Consequently, it will be easier to make an enlightened choice to meet your need: soup, pasta, rice? Cooked vegetables?... The decision is yours.

I want to draw your attention to the fact that it is a fallacy to believe that when you are hungry, it doesn't matter what you eat. Several parents have repeated this to their children when their children told them they were hungry but didn't want to eat what Mom had prepared. When it is hungry, your body is demanding one or more of the nutrients that are indispensable to its healthy functioning. If instead you give it something it doesn't need, your body will continue to demand what it is missing.

If you find it hard the first few times to carry out the exercise described above, you need only do the best you can. I can assure you that after a few days of practice, it will become easier and easier to listen to and understand what your body is demanding. It is normal that you may have difficulty if you have never taken the time to check in with your body to see what it is asking for when it lets you know that it is hungry.

To learn something new takes time and a certain amount of practice. How many people do you know who learned how to ride a bicycle instantly, how to drive a car, to dance or cook... without needing to practice for a while first? So, it is very important that you persevere and be patient with yourself. You will save yourself a lot of stress. And remember, this is about your personal well-being.

Being hungry but not knowing what to eat

At those times when you have no clue what you should eat, even when you are convinced that you are truly hungry, become aware that the same thing is happening in your life. You know you need something more in order to be happy in certain areas, but you just can't figure out right away what it is you really want. This kind of situation is most often experienced by people who have trouble establishing clear objectives for themselves, setting goals that are stimulating and energizing.

If this sounds like you, ask yourself the following question: *In ideal circumstances and if I had all the time, energy, skills and even the money necessary and if, furthermore, what I desire and choose did not bother anyone, what would I want RIGHT NOW?* Note the first answer that comes to you. This doesn't necessarily mean that this desire must manifest itself right away. But at least you will become aware of something you find exciting, makes you feel enthusiastic. All you have to do is take some initial steps that will perhaps lead to the goal you set for yourself.

Another way to become aware of what might meet one of your needs is to recall what you dreamed of being or doing when you were a child or teenager. In other words, what did you believe would really give you joy later on? There is a good chance that these un-manifested desires are an explicit part of what your heart needs. When you are in deeper contact with your real needs, you will start finding it easier to choose foods that meet the needs of your physical body.

Chapter Four

Knowing yourself through your diet

Based on what has been said so far, you become aware of the degree of love you have for yourself by observing whether you provide your physical body solely with what it needs when it needs it.

Using your diet to listen to your body is a fast and efficient way to learn whether you listen to what you need as a person. There is a difference, then, between listening to your body and listening to your needs.

Listening to your needs means taking action, giving *each* of your three "bodies" what they need, based on what you have discovered by listening to your *physical* body.

As the physical body is the tangible reflection of our two subtle – emotional and mental – bodies, it is the most reliable tool a human being has available for discovering what they refuse to see or what they find difficult to face on the emotional and intellectual level.

For example, an angry person who is convinced that everything is fine might achieve perfect self-control. But in fact, if they know how to observe and interpret their way of eating, they will also have to admit – when they see how they devour or bite into their food – that they are eating with anger.

Another person might think they are not feeling guilty about anything today, while unconsciously they are choosing to eat or drink something related to feelings of guilt. In fact, when you feel guilty about having eaten a particular food, you should use that situation to help you become aware that the real guilt is about something totally other than food. By taking the time to note what took place during the hours just prior, you will discover it is something else that you are feeling guilty about. Then, you will be able to work on the *source* of the problem and not just the food issue. If you doubt the validity of this theory and the fact that the three "bodies" reflect one another, it will be harder for you to use the methods suggested in this book. Generally speaking, a three-month test period is sufficient to determine whether a method will work for you or not. So, if you are a doubter, why not at least give yourself the opportunity to try it out? Who knows? You might get results that exceed your expectations! If my methods do not suit you, it will only have taken a total of three months of your time to find out.

Daily Journal

What I suggest you do, over the next three months, is set aside five to fifteen minutes at the end of each day to complete a daily food journal. You will find a sample journal at the end of this book. For practical purposes, this same sample is on my Web site, www.lisebourbeau.com, for you to be able to print.

As a learning tool, this journal will help you do an analysis at the end of each day. Always start with the time of day when you are making your entries, i.e., the evening, and then work your way back to when you got up to start the day. This is not about making a long list of all the ingredients in every dish, like what was in your salad or how many calories it had, but about getting a general picture of whether you are providing your body with what it needs and what prompts you to eat or drink.

To help you, here is the example of Rita, a married woman, who lives alone with her two young children and works full-time at an office.

Time	Food and beverage
9 p.m.	2 cookies and a glass of milk
6:30 p.m.	A bowl of soup A slice of bread Chicken with gravy 3 potatoes A second slice of bread 2 scoops of ice cream Tea
5:30 p.m.	2 beers Peanuts – small handful
Around 3 p.m.	2 coffees
12:30 p.m.	A hamburger Fries (large portion) A soft drink An apple croissant Coffee
11 a.m.	Coffee 2 cookies
10 a.m.	Coffee
7:30 a.m.	2 slices of toast with jam 2 coffees

When you have finished, total the number of glasses of water you drank during the day. Remember that your body needs two liters, which is the equivalent of eight glasses of

250 ml. (8 oz.), per day. A tall glass holds about 375 ml. (12 oz.).

Once you have completed the first two columns, move on to the next column where you indicate whether you were hungry or not and what made you eat or drink when you did.

During this part of the exercise, various scenarios may present themselves:

▶   You were hungry and ate only what you really wanted

▶   You were hungry and you ate indiscriminately, without checking what you needed

▶   You were hungry and you ate too much

▶   You were not really hungry and you ate for some other reason – see below.

The first step is to put a checkmark under either "Hungry" or "Not hungry". Same thing for the third column with the heading "Eat as needed". I want to remind you here that **to know whether you have listened to your need, it is important to have asked yourself beforehand whether you were hungry for warm or cold, hard or soft, sweet or not sweet.** Was it clearly what you wanted at that moment? For instance, if during the day, you start to feel hungry and the idea of eating a delicious soup makes you salivate, then that is surely what your body needs. If on the other hand, at the moment you go to eat something, you are still undecided as to what you want, that's when you need then to ask yourself the questions listed above.

I would also remind you that if you ask yourself whether you are hungry and you can't say, or it takes you a long time to answer the question, it is a pretty fair indication that you are not hungry. It's like asking yourself, *Do I want to marry X?* and it takes a while before the answer comes to you... Given the hesitation, it would surely make sense to check out your feelings before anything else and to ask yourself if you are really ready to marry.

The other six reasons for eating

There are six different motives for eating: principle, habit, emotion, gourmandise, reward and laziness. In total there are seven reasons, if we include hunger.

You are motivated by **principle** when you eat or drink, influenced by the notion of good and bad or fear. In this category you could find the following situations:

♦ Fear of wasting. Eating or drinking any substance (liquid or solid), before it goes bad or before the Best Before date. Finishing what's on your plate rather than discarding leftovers. Even finishing other people's plates. Ordering and eating the full meal offered in an all-inclusive menu, for example, bread, entree and dessert, because they are part of the deal. Choosing the cheapest food at a restaurant or market, even when it's not what you want. Depriving yourself because the price is too high, even though you know you could afford it financially.

♦ Fear of displeasing. Impossible to say no when you are offered something to eat or drink, even though you were not planning to have anything initially

♦ Fear of expressing your dislike of a certain food after you have tasted it

◆　Fear of judgment. Do what others do out of fear of what they will think or say about you

◆　Fear of consequences. Eating because you have to, without enjoyment, only because your body needs nourishment.

You are motivated by *habit* if:

◆　You often or always eat the same thing. For example, two slices of toast with peanut butter at breakfast

◆　You often or always eat at the same time

◆　You do what you learned in childhood and have done ever since, like eating three meals a day, never skipping breakfast, etc.

◆　You only stop eating when you have finished everything on your plate and you have even thoroughly cleaned it with a piece of bread.

◆　You hesitate or refuse to try a new food because you have never tasted it.

You are motivated by *emotion* if:

◆　You know you are not really hungry but something inside you prompts you to eat or drink all the same

◆　You say to yourself *I wonder what I could have to eat?* not knowing what food to choose and knowing it is not out of principle or habit that you want to eat

◆　You are angry, frustrated, hurting or lonely and you eat or drink for lack of being able to let out your feelings in some other way.

You are motivated by ***gourmandise*** (by your fondness for food) if you are motivated by one or more of your five senses:

♦ You eat or drink because it smells good

♦ You cannot help yourself because it is just so good

♦ You are attracted by a certain type of food once you have seen it, while a few minutes earlier you had not even thought about it

♦ You cannot refrain from sampling a dish once you have set eyes on it

♦ You want to eat the same thing as the person next to you.

♦ You are attracted by a food once you have touched or smelled it – you like its texture or aroma – like popcorn at the movie theatre

♦ You let yourself be influenced by what you hear, for example, when a restaurant waiter gives a glowing description of an item on the menu.

You are motivated by the need for a ***reward*** if:

♦ You have just completed a task you are proud of and therefore feel you need to eat or drink something, knowing very well it is not necessary at that particular moment

♦ You have exceeded your limits, you have worked non-stop without taking a break and you think that eating something will make you relax

♦ You feel frustrated because no one compliments you and given this situation, you eat whatever you feel like. (This situation also fits the **emotion** column.)

You are motivated by *laziness* if:

◆ You accept what someone else decides to cook for you rather than have to prepare something yourself

◆ You are home alone and so you choose a dish that doesn't require any preparation

◆ You choose not to eat rather than have to fix yourself something

◆ You buy a frozen dinner or take-out food as you leave work, planning to eat it when you get home.

I would remind you that you might also take a drink for any of the reasons contained in the six motivations listed above, even if only the word "eat" is used there. As soon as you say to yourself, *I wonder what I could have to drink?* it is important to remember that it is water that your body needs. Therefore, each time that you drink something else, you must enter it in one of the last six columns.

And it is possible that you will need to put a checkmark in more than one of the last six columns for the same food. For example, you might eat candy for reasons of both emotion and reward.

The link between the events of the day and motivation

In the column LINK, you can take the time to note whether anything special took place during the hours or minutes preceding your eating or drinking when you didn't really need to.

Let's go back to the chart showing a typical day for Rita. We can presume she will realize that the several coffees consumed are related to the stress she experiences at work and that, furthermore, she didn't really want to be at work that day. At noon, she had to deal with an emergency for her mother and, being short of time, had to buy her lunch at McDonald's. Later, the beer she had with a friend after work helped her to relax and it felt like a reward because she did not look forward to going home to the stress of her family life. The cookies she often takes in the evening are a comfort food reminding her of her happy childhood. Indeed, her mother always got a milk-and-cookies snack ready for her at bed time. As well, the two slices of toast in the morning have been part of her traditional breakfast for years. Her evening meal is something for which she may indeed have been really hungry. On the other hand, it is quite possible that she took her dessert out of habit – if she has one at the end of every meal – or just because she loves food or wants a reward.

After about a week of food journal entries (which you should make daily, preferably at the end of the day, or after each meal if you wish, and not several days later when you might forget some important information), you will find it interesting to compile the data that has accumulated. When you add up each column, you will be able to see what stands out for you in a given week. You will also see how many times you ate out of *Hunger*. It will give you the opportunity to see to what extent or what percentage of the time you are listening to your real needs, based on each of the moments in question.

Interpreting the five motivations

Here is the way to interpret the results.

EATING OUT OF PRINCIPLE OR HABIT is an indication that you allow yourself to be **too controlled or manipulated by your beliefs**. These come mainly from your education or what you learned as a child or adolescent. It is the past, then, that is directing your life. Several fears prevent you from listening to your intuition and your genuine needs. As a result you must surely be letting numerous interesting occasions pass you by. Moreover, it is very likely that you are among those who resist new ideas or suggestions offered by others.

In short, the person who does not take the time to ask themselves if they are hungry and who eats out of principle or habit is one who allows the notions of good and bad, should and shouldn't, appropriate and inappropriate to direct them. The ego is directing the stomach. This type of person also has trouble pleasing themselves or tasting life's pleasures, believing it is wrong to do so until all chores and tasks have been completed. They may also believe other people's enjoyment should come before their own. This type of person will often buy items in a store based on price rather than on what they really want.

EATING OUT OF EMOTION is an indication that your emotions are much stronger – consciously or not – than you want to admit. You are the kind of person who tries to separate yourself from your feelings. You may be experiencing anger, frustration, disappointment, sadness or loneliness, but you try as much as possible to avoid going too deep and feeling the pain associated with your emotions. It is a strat-

74

egy many people use, thinking they will suffer less that way. It is important to remember that when you experience emotions, it means you have a lot of expectations. **You expect other people to show you love or affection the way you want them to.** Since no one is responsible for the happiness of others, your expectations are often unmet and every time this happens, you try to fill the inner emptiness with food. *A priori*, we often have strong emotional reactions when we confuse LOVING and PLEASING.

EATING OUT OF GOURMANDISE is an indication that your senses are psychologically not satisfied. Generally speaking, you let yourself be influenced in life by your senses, by what you see and hear and by what you sense in others. In most people, this is because they feel responsible for the happiness of others. You often feel obliged to do something for people with problems. You should know that people who think they are responsible for the good fortune or misfortune of others often feel guilty. How much this is reflected in the way they eat will correspond to the degree of guilt they feel toward others. Moreover, it is very likely that you find it hard to let those you love make up their own minds about things, especially when you do not agree with them. **Your happiness depends on the happiness of others and this creates emptiness in your heart that you try to fill with food, instead of learning to fill it by meeting your true needs.**

EATING TO REWARD YOURSELF indicates that you might be someone who asks a lot of yourself, asking things that are beyond your limits. **Possibly, you are perfectionist by nature and you wait till you have accomplished something extraordinary before you reward yourself.** It appears you often wait till others acknowledge you, congratulate you or pay you compliments. Since there is no one on this earth whose mandate it is to ensure the happiness of others, most of us experience disappointment and even bitterness in the wake of our unfulfilled expectations.

You might also be someone who does not savour the rewards you do give yourself, putting too much emphasis on everything you still have to do.

EATING OUT OF LAZINESS indicates that you are probably more dependent on others than you think. When you are in the presence of those you love, you must be a different person than when you are alone. You believe you must act in accordance with their choices. This means that you don't think you are important enough. The presence of other people gives you a false sense of importance. **You do not believe sufficiently in your worth as a person to take the time to listen to your own needs.** It may also be that when someone fixes something delicious for you, it feels like you are receiving a form of your mother's love and it reminds you of that particular kind of happiness or lack of it.

When you discover, by completing this journal, that you have not listened to your needs very well, be sure not to start feeling guilty. The main goal of this exercise is to get to know yourself and not to add another stress into your life. In the final two chapters you will learn what attitude to develop so you can live this experience with acceptance.

Compulsion

I have not assigned a specific place in the food journal for you to note down whether sometimes you eat or drink out of COMPULSION. To clarify what I mean by this, it is a term used when a person starts ingesting a food or a beverage and then simply cannot stop anymore. At first they start because they are hungry or for any other reason, like emotion, and suddenly they don't know how to stop. For example, they might devour an entire tub of ice cream, or a whole bag of chips, or all the chocolates in a box. Another person might feel like eating spaghetti, take a portion that would normally be sufficient, but then without realizing it, take another and another. What began as a desire to satisfy hunger ends up becoming a compulsion. This attitude is frequently encountered at dessert time when mostly we are no longer hungry but still wolf down several portions of dessert.

This situation is an indication of a great lack of self-love and self-esteem. If you sometimes find yourself in this type of situation, it is important to ask yourself, as soon as you become aware of it, what has just happened to you in the last few hours to make you look down on yourself in this way. It's as if your heart is so empty of self-love, you try to fill it with food and you realize that even if you keep eating till your stomach feels full, your heart will keep feeling just as empty. However, all it needs is for you to pay it some sincere compliments and for you to recognize all that is good and beautiful about you both on the inside and on the outside.

Those who are most inclined to have this type of compulsion are those who systematically reject themselves, who are far too demanding of themselves. Nothing is ever perfect enough for their taste. Moreover, their level of self-love is so low that they are convinced that no one in the world could love them for who they are. They are therefore eternally dissatisfied, no matter what others say or do for them.

If you become aware, while you are filling out your food journal, that you act out of compulsion, it is important to note it in the column called LINK.

Link analysis

This last column, where you note down all the connections you are able to make between the incidents of each day and your way of eating, is very important. It allows you to do a kind of in-depth analysis. This does not mean you have to fix everything as you go along. On the contrary, becoming conscious of everything so rapidly allows you to make improvements in your life that may quite often appear without you even realizing it.

When you realize that most of the food or drink you consumed during the day was not taken out of genuine hunger, you know that you were not in charge of yourself, that you were not listening to your real needs and you did not love yourself enough. This observation indicates that you had to try to control yourself or someone else during the day and that, accordingly, you lost control over how you eat. If you refer to the first chapter of this book, you will be able to make the link with one of your wounds that was activated, to which you then reacted. The stage that automatically follows this reaction is a lapse into control mode, which prevents us from being our own masters.

Let's return to the example of Rita, described above. When she observes how many coffees she had during the day and that she did not really feel like going to work that day, it can help her become aware of certain realities: Her work offers her little stimulation now and is no longer sufficiently challenging; she has learned all she can from this job... Even if she doesn't make a decision when she notes this in her journal in the evening, she is already on the road to finding a solution. Does she need to find another job? Does she need to meet with her boss to share her experience and her lack of motivation so that they can determine together whether a different set of responsibilities might motivate her more? Does she need to find stimulation outside of work, an exciting hobby or sport?

It is thus possible that she will become conscious of the role of her wound of injustice, which until now has blocked her awareness of her dissatisfaction at work, because she was afraid of making a wrong decision. Or perhaps it is her wound of abandonment, letting her believe that her husband would be very disappointed if she left her job even though he earns a good salary, and she may be afraid of displeasing him.

As you can see, noting everything down as you go along helps a great deal with being able to see things as they really are and to put them into perspective. Gradually, with the help of several clues presented to you day after day, it becomes much easier to recognize your genuine needs and to listen to them better.

I would like to remind you that it is extremely important to fill out the daily journal at the end of each day and to compile the data at the end of a week. The use of this tool constitutes your best method. It is preferable to enter the whole week, using both the front and back of a sheet. It is the outcome of the compiled data that will help you to really know yourself. Be assured that, each day, as you log information in your journal, you will become conscious of several aspects of yourself that would have been hard to discover otherwise.

At the end of a week, you will be made more aware of the current strong influences in your life by noting what prompted you to eat when you were not listening to your needs. Remind yourself, especially at the beginning, to check which wounds were activated the most, by referring to the examples of control mentioned in the first chapter of this book.

You will see that sometimes you are controlling yourself, sometimes you want to control others and at other times, you let others control you. These three control modes indicate that you are not using your innate power to create your life. You are trying instead to have power over others or allowing others to take your power away from you.

Gradually, as you make more and more connections between your dietary habits and the control mechanisms reflected there, you will start to understand what is hiding in all those times you eat out of principle, habit, emotion, fondness for food, reward or laziness.

When you notice that in a particular week you have eaten much more often out of hunger, you will be happy to note that you have been doing a better job of listening to your body. You will then become aware that your wounds were not activated as often, that you were more yourself –

an indication of how much you are growing in self-love and self-acceptance.

The first two or three weeks will be the toughest, especially if you find it hard to discipline yourself. However, the fact that you are reading this book shows that you are prepared to try new experiences. Find a way to motivate yourself to complete the journal every evening. It might be the joy that will come from being more in charge of your life, or the joy of returning to a healthier you or to your ideal weight. Or you might think of a way to reward yourself at the end of the week after completing your journal. For example, something to eat or drink or to buy for yourself that you don't really need, or going out just for your own enjoyment. It doesn't matter what the reward is, it's something you deserve, so take the time to savour it. I want to clarify here that whatever you eat or drink WITHOUT GUILT, WITH LOVE, cannot do you any harm. In fact, the reality may well be the very opposite…

It might even be a good idea to put out a sign or some other object to make you think of filling out the journal. After two or three weeks, it will become a habit and then it will be much easier. Moreover, you will be so thrilled by the discoveries you make about yourself that you will feel more and more inclined to follow through on your commitment.

You must sustain this habit for a minimum of three months, in order to obtain a clear and precise picture of what is going on in your deepest self. Then, you can stop for a few months, but it would nevertheless be an excellent idea to start up again a little later. For example, three months of journal keeping, three months break, followed by three months of journal keeping and again a three-month break, and so forth. This will allow you to see if you are able to keep on asking yourself the right questions, to know if your REALLY are HUNGRY and what your body needs, without having to remind yourself every evening to fill out a journal.

To conclude this chapter, I have one last suggestion that might help smokers get to know themselves better. They could enter into their journal what motivates them to smoke. One person shared with me that she discovered new aspects of herself by doing this exercise.

Just writing everything down this way at the end of each day is an enormous help toward accepting oneself. The secret is to write everything down without any judgment, and to remind yourself that all you want is to know yourself better.

Chapter Five

Your dietary habits and your weight

Is it possible, in your opinion, that something other than your diet could be causing your excess weight? Indeed, it is possible. The objective of this chapter is to help you realize how much a person's inner attitude affects the choices they make, with respect to foods that do or do not cause weight gain.

You have surely noticed among those around you that there are several people who eat what they want when they want and still manage to keep their weight the same, year after year. You have probably seen others who, as soon as they indulge in the slightest excess in their diet, start to put on weight. You might hear the explanation, *Yes, but that's because of their genetic makeup.* My reply to that would be, *Is it possible that there is a link between the genes these people chose before birth and their current life pattern?*

I have been able to observe this reality in thousands of people since 1981, the year I became conscious of the connection between inner attitude and weight. As I write this book, I have been verifying for twenty-eight years the accuracy of my synthesis and I never tire of observing and discovering new data. I am happy to note that in the last several years, we have been hearing more and more people – doctors, nutritionists, psychologists, etc. – talk about this link between inner attitude and weight.

My comments are not intended to give the impression that diet plays no part in the problem of being overweight. It is in fact true that, when we are not ourselves, we do not listen to the needs of our body and are inclined to give it foods it does not need, which it must then "store". The aim of this chapter is primarily to develop awareness of how much influence inner attitude has on weight problems.

So then, what is this attitude that has such a significant influence on a person's weight? For starters, it is imperative to accept the fact that we all have a natural biological weight that is right for us. Insurance companies were the first to establish an ideal weight table as a criteria for determining whether a person is considered obese or not. This table is now used by everyone interested in the question of weight. I support this approach too. I agree that a great many people weigh far more than their natural weight and this table can assist them by offering a realistic and objective guideline. For those who are interested, you can consult the Internet to learn how to calculate your Body Mass Index (BMI), which will help you find out whether you are suffering from obesity or from being overweight.

I am convinced that if all children learned from their earliest years how important their inner attitude is, there would be very little obesity on this planet. Of course, there would be some people who are slimmer than others but, if everyone adopted a healthy inner attitude from the start, they would find their natural weight much easier to maintain.

It is my pleasure to be able to testify to the truth of this, based on what I have observed in my children and grandchildren. In fact, at the time when I became aware of the link between inner attitude and weight, my children were aged 13, 15 and 19. Today, twenty-eight years later, my three children have still never deviated from their natural weight. Of course, their bodies have changed with the years, but that is a natural phenomenon, in keeping also with how our attitude changes. I have noticed as well that my grandchildren, like most other children of the "new age", listen to their bodies naturally and it is impossible to make them eat food they don't want when they aren't hungry.

Our inner attitude is affected and influenced by the wounds with which we are born. All of us have at least four of the five wounds mentioned in Chapter One but I have noticed that most people are influenced more by one wound than another when it comes to their dietary habits. Everything depends on how they were emotionally nourished by their mother and what they retained of that during their childhood with respect to food.

In the natural order of things, it is the mother who feeds her child. Therefore, she has an enormous influence on the decision her child will make, to like or not like this maternal gesture. In reality, she will feed her child according to the desire or interest the child expresses, which will of course be in keeping with the wounds its soul needs to work on, but she will do this unknowingly. This is why a mother feeds each of her children in a different way that is particular to them. Moms who have several children will tell you that they act differently with each of their children because over time, they change their habits from one child to the next. But most of them are not aware that it is rather what they need to learn – the mom in relation to this child and this child in relation to its mother – that strongly influences their way of feeding each of their children.

Children who need to work on their wound of humiliation, for example, will attract a mother who likewise needs to work on accepting this wound, so that both of them can engage in the process of healing. This immutable law, the fact that everything we attract comes from inside ourselves, exists everywhere in the world. No one can escape it, and the same is true for all the wounds. **We attract the people and situations our soul needs, in order to learn true love and unconditional acceptance.**

If you have completely changed the way you eat or you notice you have suddenly gained or lost a lot of weight, it shows that another wound has been activated. Whatever you went through was so major that it got the upper hand. Let's take a look together at which wound it was that affected you.

The influence of the wound of rejection on weight

The inner attitude of a person whose body carries this wound is I am nothing… *I must take up as little space as possible… even if I disappear, no one will notice… physical pleasure does not interest me… I'd rather nourish my mind…* With this kind of inner attitude, it is impossible for this person to put on weight, seeing as they want to disappear, take up as little room as possible, make themselves almost "invisible". This person is inclined to eat very little and, even if they eat several times a day or choose foods that are supposed to be fattening, nothing really affects their weight. Furthermore, these people, being of nervous temperament, generally have a fast metabolism, which is another reason why they do not gain weight. On the other hand, their digestive system has to work harder.

We find in this category of people those who rejected their mother's way of nourishing them, not just physically, but also and especially, emotionally. They did not feel loved and accepted for who they were and this was probably true from the moment they were born.

These people specialize in denial. For instance, they will pretend and even try to make themselves believe that they never eat sugar, even if they do. They will state that they do not like this or that, without realizing that this "denying themselves nourishment" comes from the fact that they do not take the time to really taste their food. Moreover, the wound of rejection is very often at the root of a drug or alcohol problem, but these people refuse to admit that they might have that kind of problem because they are so clever at denying reality.

The influence of the wound of abandonment on weight

The inner attitude of a person who suffers from the wound of abandonment could be reflected in various statements, such as: *I need more attention and support. I never get enough.* Those who hold this attitude of "never enough" are the type of person who can consume a huge quantity of food to fill up, without, however, gaining any weight. These people have often received a lot of attention from their mother or from whoever played that role, but as they believe they never received enough, and have always held on to their sense of deprivation, they are unable to ac-knowledge this fact.

They are always trying to fill this void with the parent of the opposite sex, convinced that if this parent would prove their love for them by showing them attention, it would indicate that they are lovable and deserving of attention. They also believe that getting attention is the only way to feel filled with love. When they are not getting the attention or support that they desire, they feel abandoned. So, they set their heart on eating, and are able to do so without gain-ing a single pound, as they adhere to the belief of "not enough". These abuses affect their digestive system, as happens with those suffering from rejection.

The influence of the wound of humiliation on weight

The inner attitude of people who suffer from this wound will differ from that of people with the other wounds. Why? Because everything that concerns satisfying the senses takes on a strong feeling of importance and pleasure for these people. In fact, those who are born with this wound need to learn to savour fully the pleasures afforded by their five physical senses WITHOUT FEELING GUILTY and especially without thinking that it makes them unworthy of God's love.

Already at a very young age, such persons attract situa-tions that will be humiliating to them, when they are too eager for sensual pleasure. However, the lesson they learn very soon is that it is not good to be sensual. They attract negative, critical, behaviour from their educators to help them become aware that they actually believe the same thing. But it turns out to be a false belief.

If you are among those who suffer from this wound of humiliation, you must certainly remember several incidents when your parents or educators scolded you, especially about physical things. For example, if you soiled your clothes or ate a lot more than the others or attracted looks by your sensual movements. You must, furthermore, be a very spiritual person, with the intention of pleasing God in every way possible. It is those who carry this wound who are the most afraid of being unworthy before God. They are also afraid of being punished in general.

Let us note for example what happens in the United States. We know it is a country where the word *God* is used a lot in conversations. Even the presidents want the people to know that they are believers, or religious people who attend mass every Sunday, for instance. I understand that Americans are the only ones to have a currency with the word *God* inscribed on it. *In God we trust.* They are also well known for frequently saying *God bless you.*

This same country is known to have the highest percentage of obese people in the world. As well, for the majority of them, God and religion are very important in their life. As a result, they experience a great deal of guilt at the idea of seeking pleasure through physical consumption or through the senses.

The inner attitude of people who suffer from humiliation is *Here I go eating something fattening again... What a pig I am... I just love food too much... I should stop, or else I'll just get fatter... I'm so big already, so what do a few more pounds matter... I'll never manage to lose weight, might as well enjoy it.* What most people don't realize is that it is because of their huge guilt and their disparaging thoughts about themselves that they are unable to experience genuine pleasure.

To sum up, these people learned when they were young that it was not good to enjoy their food, it was egotistical to think about their own pleasure first. They were taught that they should always be concerned for the happiness and pleasure of others before their own. Having continued to behave accordingly after that and receiving nothing in exchange, they make up for it with food.

That is why people with this wound, of all the wounds, are those who will gain weight the most easily and the most rapidly. It is not so much what they consume, but their attitude toward it, that makes all the difference. Contrary to those with the first two wounds, this group maintains the inner attitude of "too much". They will say or think *I'm eating too much again. I have to stop myself.*

It also explains why they often think they're not eating more than anyone else and are surprised at their excess weight. On the other hand, being deeply attracted by the pleasure of the senses, these people frequently lose control when it comes to food. Most of the time when this happens, they hide, as they are overcome by shame. There is also the fact that the more often they tell themselves that they MUST stop eating, the more they eat. This phenomenon is explained in greater detail in the final chapter. Remember, though, that there are in this world some very tiny people who can eat as much as they want, and still not gain a single pound.

When people with the wound of humiliation gain weight, their body becomes rounder and they take on a tub-like appearance. They don't need to be very overweight for the roundness to be noticed We will learn in the next two chapters how to turn this situation around, how to let go of the guilt and how to find renewed pleasure in eating, without, however, gaining weight.

The influence of the wound of betrayal on weight

The inner attitude of those who suffer from betrayal is *I don't want to miss anything... I want to taste everything... I can do whatever I want... I don't have to follow other people's rules, or my body's rules... I'm the one in control here, not other people.* When they were young, these people often felt controlled as to how they ate. It was their parents, among others, who decided for them. They try to make up for this as soon as they can. This is the type of child who, when their parents are away, will eat precisely the foods the parents do not allow. I remember one of my sons, who would not only eat what he wanted during my absence, but would settle himself in my beautiful new arm-chair in the living room to have it. This, even though he knew my rule of no eating in this freshly decorated room. When I got back, I found the plate with crumbs on the floor beside the chair. At that time, I didn't know why he would leave such traces and bring upon himself inevitable punishment. I told him it was not a very intelligent thing to do, as he knew full well I would have to punish him. If at least he had tidied everything away before my return, I would never have known that he had disobeyed me. Today, on the other hand, I am able to understand why he acted the way he did. He was in fact letting me know that I could never control him completely. From my own personal growth journey and experiences, I now know that children who are controlled too severely by their parents are influenced by their wound of betrayal to disobey in order to have their own worth acknowledged. Once he was an adult and no longer subject to my control, he decided to eat junk food as often as he wanted. It was his way of letting me know that he didn't have to follow my advice on healthy eating anymore.

Children who have been controlled in this way have not received the emotional nourishment that should normally have satisfied their needs. The love they received from their parents was too possessive and controlling. They were raised by parents who loved them according to what they thought was best, according to what they themselves had learned from their own parents and not according to the needs of the child.

As an adult, this type of person often adds too much salt or spice to their food. We know it is because they do not really taste the food itself. They will try to prolong tasting until they have satisfied their taste buds, which seek to be satisfied by the taste of each food.

Moreover, as this person often eats rapidly, their brain is prevented from receiving the message in time that their body is no longer hungry. This type of person refuses, most of the time, to be controlled by anyone, let alone by their body.

People suffering from the wound of betrayal do not listen to their body, as seen from the fact that they eat much more often than necessary. So then, they feel guilty because they know and feel that they have eaten too much. And this is the guilt that makes them gain weight.

In women, it is especially around their hips and stomach that the weight will tend to settle, while in men it goes to the shoulders and stomach. Due to this generally more ro-bust appearance of the upper body, men who are heavy will unconsciously try to show how strong and capable they are. It makes us tend to call them strong rather than fat or obese.

The influence of the wound of injustice on weight

The person suffering from this wound has an inner atti-tude that says, *I have to be perfect in everything, especially where it concerns my actions and my appearance... I am not allowed to cheat... I must always pay attention to what I eat in order to maintain a perfect body...* This is the per-son who imposes the most control on him or herself. As they are very demanding of themselves, these people will not be able to tolerate it when they put on a few pounds. They check their weight constantly and go on a diet as soon as it fluctuates the least little bit. Many of them are on a diet almost their entire life, because they are so afraid of gaining weight. Every time they cheat on their self-imposed diet, they feel extremely guilty and then promise them-selves they will never to do it again. They achieve success for a period of time, but as we all have our limits, the day comes when they find it just about impossible to maintain perfect control.

They will try to camouflage their weaknesses concern-ing food as much as possible and will refuse to admit that their losses of control happen constantly and on a regular basis. Furthermore, people for whom this type of behaviour is typical do not realize that these losses of control with respect to food are mostly caused by the control they are exercising in other areas, ever seeking perfection in what they do.

Let's take the example of an ordinary day when a person has imposed several tasks on themselves that are well beyond their normal limits. It is highly likely that at the end of that day they will want to reward themselves and that they will lose control over what they eat or drink. *I really deserve this*, they will think to themselves. Indeed, merit is very important to those who suffer from injustice. They will have been unaware of their needs throughout the entire day, because of their fear of not being perfect or of being judged as lazy or negligent. This is why, after controlling the little voice inside them all day was trying to tell them they had reached their limit, this type of person loses control.

As food is a reflection of what is going on with our inner life, it offers us an excellent way of recognizing the times when we have been too hard on ourselves.

This type of person ends up putting on weight over the years but, in general, it will be distributed uniformly throughout the body. In fact, it is the guilt experienced by this person that makes them gain weight. They put themselves back on a diet and the vicious circle starts all over again. These people show the same intolerance toward others who gain weight as they do toward themselves.

Summary

In summary, we can conclude that when the wounds of rejection and abandonment are the ones activated the most, these people *cannot* gain weight, no matter how much food they consume. Why? Because of their motive for eating. Those who see that they *are* gaining weight must therefore be influenced by one of the other three wounds, humiliation, betrayal or injustice. The weight is distributed differently in the body, according to the wound in question.

On the influence of the different wounds, when you identify with one of the above descriptions, you will discover which wound is the most activated and the least accepted in your present life. It is quite common to be influenced by more than one wound during the same period. For example, a masochistic person – suffering from the wound of humiliation – may, for a week, be unable to stop their desire to eat a lot of cake and, after that, go on a diet. The decision to impose a diet on oneself is influenced by their rigid side – activated by the wound of injustice.

I would like to remind you that the primary reason why anyone gains weight is guilt, which is then followed by non-acceptance of oneself. The way this plays out with respect to food is the same as what is happening in other areas of one's life. The less you listen to your dietary needs, the less you are listening to your needs in life generally. This is why you feel so guilty.

This does not mean that people who do not gain weight do not feel guilty. Far from it. However, that guilt will affect their body in a different way. Instead of gaining weight, they will have health problems or accidents. When their guilt affects their weight, it is their rigid, controlling or masochistic side that has taken over.

We will see in the last chapter how to transform this guilt into responsibility.

Should we weigh ourselves or not?

It is the person trying to be perfect who will step on that scale the most, sometimes even every day. People have often asked me whether it's a good idea to weigh yourself on a regular basis. As I am among those carrying a big wound of injustice in this life, I can easily understand those who find it hard to watch their body gaining weight, especially if they have never had a weight problem before.

In my case, this happened when I reached menopause and I must admit that the bathroom scale was not helpful. As soon as I saw my weight go up, I felt guiltier about satisfying my hunger, and believed I should deny myself. When the scale showed a drop in weight, it was as if it was giving me permission to "spoil" myself a little more. So, if this instrument has the same effect on you, I would reply right off the bat that it is probably not a good idea to check your weight too often. I know people who are so influenced by the numbers they see on that scale, that it can affect their mood for the entire day.

On the other hand, if you want to know your weight occasionally, without letting it have a major influence on the way you eat or on your self-esteem, then keeping a scale in your home certainly won't do you any harm. Generally, our clothes are a clear enough indicator of what is going on, without our having to check our weight fluctuations incessantly.

Joining support groups
for weight loss

Another question I am frequently asked is: *Is it a good idea to join one of the numerous groups established for the purpose of helping people lose weight?* I cannot answer this question for you. I would suggest instead that you ask yourself the following questions, which will help you to find your own answer: *Do I feel guilty when I deviate from the suggested program or when I am weighed at a meeting and if I have put on a pound during the week?... Do I feel better after these meetings?... Do their meal suggestions help me to eat in a healthier way, without feeling that I am always hungry?* If you perceive that on the whole, being a member of one of these groups provides you with significantly more pleasant than unpleasant consequences, well then, why not go ahead? It is important to develop the ability to discern clearly in life and especially to take decisions that are intelligent and appropriate for oneself. We must recognize that nothing is right for everyone, regardless of what field we are talking about. Each of us has different needs. We need to make our own choices, take our own decisions, and not decide on the basis of an experience that has been good for someone else.

If you do not find the answers to the above questions useful, it might be wise to try a group for at least three months before joining. After that, it should be easier for you to determine what is best for you.

Awareness and
weight gain

There is a phenomenon that appears sometimes in our workshops, especially among women. We have observed that when a participant begins to be more aware of her beliefs, wounds and fears, she starts to put on a few pounds. This phenomenon seems particularly prevalent among those with the wound of injustice. Why is this?

It's because they have been applying control mechanisms so much up until now that they have finally reached a point where they realize they cannot continue that way. If you fit this group, definitely do not get discouraged. It means that your natural weight had not yet been reached. Your body is no longer so subject to your control. It is now being allowed to find its natural state. Consequently, a rather major adjustment will be required on your part in this situation.

You may gain (or lose) weight well beyond your natural state. This is probably because you were no longer able to sustain that level of control. The decision – often made unconsciously – to transform one attitude into another, can take you to extremes. You have become incapable of controlling your body. It's as if a pendulum has swung way over to one side and then, when you let yourself go, it swings right over to the opposite side. It needs the opportunity to go back and forth until it can finally settle in the middle. The same will happen to you if you trust your body. You simply have to give yourself the time to reach that stage.

Sudden weight gain

It also happens often that people say they have gained forty or even sixty pounds in the space of a few months. This sudden weight gain is the result of a major – physical and psychological – shock, triggered by a situation that involved more than one wound and was not accepted.

When we compensate with food, following a shock like this, it's because we feel guilty about the situation. We are eating our food out of a sense of blame-taking. It is moreover this great guilt that is making us gain so much weight. It is our body's way of trying to draw our attention – dramatically (as easily seen in a mirror) – to the fact that it is high time we learned to love ourselves more and to give ourselves the right to be human, with all our weaknesses and limitations.

Chapter Six

Letting go
and your diet

I have mentioned several times since the beginning of this book that we cannot dissociate our three "bodies" – the physical, emotional and mental. Accordingly, when you lack energy, it is because one of those bodies is undernourished. In this chapter, I will describe concrete methods you can use, especially as applied to the physical body, that will automatically have an impact on the other two bodies, that is, on your inner attitude and, therefore, on your behaviour. The next chapter will deal more with the spiritual aspect: your heart and your soul.

The ideal weight

To begin with, it is important to be clear about what is meant by ideal weight. I often hear the question: *How do I know what my ideal weight is?* Only you can determine and, especially, feel this. Only your body knows what the natural weight is for you. Natural doesn't mean normal. Certain people will have to be large all their life, if it is part of their life journey. They may need to learn to love themselves that way – and so it is their natural weight.

Your body will return to its natural weight as soon as it stops being afraid you're going to make it endure famine. Yes, that is how your body perceives the deprivations you impose on it. Even if you are not following a specific diet and you are not aware of depriving yourself or of being afraid of eating too much, your body perceives your intention. I would remind you that, on average, human beings are conscious of barely ten percent of what is going on inside them. The body hears the little voice in your head that often thinks *I ate too much again; I have to discipline myself... have more self-control... I have to use more moderation.* And then, when you call yourself all sorts of names because you think you have been lacking in self-control, or as you look at your body, or after indulging in too large a meal, it hears that too.

So, when you want to impose deprivation on your body, it is quite normal for it to react by stocking up on reserves. It reacts exactly the way you would in any other field. Suppose that you find out that in a few months you will have to give up your job for six months, and that there will be no alternative source of income during that time. Surely you would react by setting aside enough money to get you through those months. Wouldn't that be a normal reaction? Well, your body experiences the same thing. It is making provision.

When you transform your inner attitude and start loving yourself more, I can assure you that your body will feel it and will gently guide itself toward its natural weight, which will vary, upwards or downwards, with the individual.

Only people on a strict diet achieve rapid weight loss. What most of them don't know is that on a low cal diet, the body becomes deficient in certain calories that provide necessary energy; consequently, it has to look to the muscle tissue for an alternative source of that energy. However, when you listen to your body instead of depriving it, it will return to its natural weight and only the fat will fall away.

It is when there starts to be muscle loss that the body feels it is undergoing famine. It becomes anxious, knowing that with weakened muscles, it cannot function in its natural state. Now it enters a struggle because, applying its great intelligence, it always does everything in its power to maintain its well-being. I'm not really telling you anything new, am I? You have no doubt observed this phenomenon many times when you have hurt yourself. Without you having to instruct your body in any way whatsoever, it sets everything in motion to start the process of healing the wound or the illness, as required.

It has been shown scientifically that when a person goes on a diet, their metabolism slows down more and more. Our metabolism's job is to consume the energy needed for, among other things, the proper functioning of our brain, our heart and our respiratory and digestive systems and the maintenance of our body heat at a constant temperature. So, when the metabolism is slowed down like that, we digest more slowly. That's why people on a diet get the impression that the least amount of food makes them gain weight. It's simply the body doing its work.

The decision to put yourself on a diet is unnatural because it is motivated by fear. To be natural is to be yourself, to let yourself be guided by the needs of your own nature; it's loving yourself every instant. Since we know that the body will do everything it can to find the balance and energy necessary to return to its natural state, we are not surprised to realize that a weight loss diet can only achieve temporary results. Statistics show unequivocally that 90%

of people who lose weight as the result of a diet regain that weight and a few additional pounds during the following two years. The ones who maintain their weight are those who are always on a diet. This is why the weight loss industry is one of the biggest and most lucrative in the world. It involves starting over and over again.

As far as fatty tissue is concerned, it is the principal site where the body stores toxins. In David Servan-Schreiber's book, *Anticancer* – a book I strongly recommend – he talks about Dr. Davis, who heads a "cancer and the environment" research centre at Pittsburg University. Dr. Davis maintains that our excess fat is like a "toxic waste dump" for the body. Therefore it is preferable to lose fat, not muscle, when we slim down. It will help you get rid of harmful toxins. This is also why a doctor will always advise people who are particularly heavy, and are sick, that they need to lose weight. Doctors know this is a determining factor for health and healing.

Daily needs are different

Depending on the nature of our daily activities, the body expends more or less energy. For instance, it you are doing heavy physical work, your body's dietary needs will be different than when you spend a good part of your day seated and doing only moderate physical work, or lounging around and watching TV. Another relevant fact: if you perspire a lot, your body will need that much more salt and water.

If your work demands considerable intellectual effort, you will need a greater supply of calories. Did you know that the brain, although it constitutes only 2% of your weight, by itself requires 50% of the glucose you consume? It needs at least the equivalent of 500 calories of glucose a day, while the muscles, which generally represent 50% of your body mass, only demand 20% of your body's energy.

This is why it is so important to listen to what your body needs. If your body is asking for sweet foods, it's what you must give it. If you follow the suggestions given in the earlier chapters, you will gradually become more aware of whether it is really your body asking for the sugar or whether it is a desire influenced by emotions.

But it doesn't matter! Starting now, why not give yourself the right to eat what pleases you? Tell your body that you are in the process of learning to listen to it, even if you cannot be sure one hundred percent of the time that you have understood correctly what it needs. Ask your body also to be patient enough with you to eliminate whatever it does not need at present. Reassure it that very likely it will soon have less extra work to do, as you start to be more aware of your needs.

The important thing is to remember that each day is different, that you may need two large meals one day and five small meals the next.

Respecting the needs
of others

If you live in a family or with others and you are in charge of the meals, it is very important to remember that you will never find everyone being hungry at the same time, to the same degree, and with the same needs.

Yes, but I'm not a servant. I can't after all make four different meals!!! Isn't that what you will say? If you only knew how often I have heard that said! However, I assure you that all the members of one family can learn to each listen to their own needs without it being all that complicated.

My children were teenagers when I started to apply this method. Prior to that, I used to insist that everyone eat what I had prepared, repeating to them the sentence in the above paragraph. Obviously, given their different tastes, they would often make a scene. When they refused to eat the dishes I had prepared for them, I would get upset. I would get frustrated because of the great amount of time wasted preparing such a good meal, since they hardly appreciated it.

I finally realized I was operating out of the same beliefs my mother had held:

- ▶ We must eat three meals a day to be healthy;

- ▶ Preparing good meals for those we love, feeding them well, is a way of letting them know how much we love them.

So, when they refused to eat at the so-called normal time or turned down their nose at the special dishes I made for them or wanted to skip a meal, I was convinced their health would suffer. Wanting to be the perfect mother, I was afraid of being judged a bad mom if they were to get sick because of not eating. There you have a good example of control caused by the wound of injustice. Besides being afraid of not being a perfect mother, I felt being a mom was a thankless job and that I was being unfairly treated as it was impossible to make everybody happy.

At the same time, this type of situation was making me slide into my wound of rejection because of that second belief. It was as if they were rejecting my love.

I had been experiencing this from the time I got married. It's not a co-incidence that I married a man whose mother hardly cooked; he wasn't used to all those different dishes. You can guess the rest. He would sit down at the table, stare at his plate for a few seconds and then blurt out, *I'm sorry, I'm not hungry*. It was like a knife went through my heart. I insisted he at least taste it. After forcing himself to eat a few mouthfuls, he got up from the table and as soon as he thought no one was looking, after the meal, he rifled through the cupboards looking for something else to eat.

The children repeated this scenario quite often too. It took me many years to become aware that I had to learn to let go rather than let my beliefs direct my life.

When I finally decided to adopt a new attitude, to stop dramatizing and to adopt a different kind of behaviour, after I became aware of the importance of listening to one's needs, everything went very well, much better in fact than I could have anticipated. I continued to prepare meals at normal times without really worrying about their tastes or whether they were hungry. Whoever wasn't hungry no longer felt obliged to eat, knowing clearly that they had the option of taking their meal (cold) an hour or two later. I realized that chicken and vegetables contain just as much nutrition when they are cold as when they are warm. If one of them felt like eating something different, they could go and check out the fridge or else make themselves a sandwich.

I will admit, though, that these situations only arose once or twice a week. Most of the time, my family was keen to eat what I had prepared because I had let go.

Yes, but who knows what they're going to eat if I let them eat whatever they want. Isn't that your reaction? Well, if that's what you're afraid of, I have a question for you: Who buys the food that comes into your house? All you have to do is make sure you have only good healthy food in your kitchen and then it won't matter what they choose, it will always be nutritious for them. You will see how much easier you have made your life, by letting go this way.

So, I told my children, who were in their early teens at that time,, that they could buy themselves anything they wanted from the convenience store – candy, chocolate, pop, chips, etc. – out of their weekly allowance. At first they were eager to go and get things I didn't necessarily approve of. However, I took the time to explain clearly to them the harmful effects of some of those products, but emphasized that in the end, they were in charge of their own bodies and that from now on it would be up to them to decide whether to harm their body or not and they would have to take the consequences. Responsibility for their body was now theirs, with no intervention from me. Gradually and of their own accord, they bought less and less junk food, preferring to use their money for other things.

When we take responsibility and know we have to assume unpleasant consequences, it goes a long way toward helping us not feel guilty, as well as make wiser food choices. It becomes easier for the body to co-operate with us.

I also want to draw your attention to the difference between the needs of women and men. Your partner does not have the same basic needs as you do. A man's metabolism is 15-20% faster than a woman's. As men are generally equipped with a larger frame and stature, they are able to absorb more calories.

Most couples are inclined to eat the same thing, because the person preparing the meal thinks they have to produce two identical dinners. This is another habit that could use some revision.

Are you one of those people who want to show their love by preparing wonderful meals? If you are, it is very likely you have trouble saying no to people who offer you food – which used to be the case with me. If someone insists that you eat or drink something, one approach that seems to work very well is to say *No thank you, not just now, perhaps later* or *let me think about it*. This is a new habit worth adopting and developing. Later on, it will be easy for you to simply say, *No thank you, I'm not hungry* or *I don't want any, thanks,* without having to offer an explanation. You will have reached the final stage when you can just say, *No, thank you.* You will then be communicating such self-assurance that no one will dare to insist. They will inevitably feel that your NO is genuine and sincere.

Remember that what you experience regarding the way you nourish yourself helps you know yourself in other spheres of your life. By learning to say *No thank you* in relation to food, you are learning a skill you can also apply in other areas. There will always be people who will try to convince you to change your mind and bring you round to what they want in other spheres of your life. It is certainly not with the intention to hurt you, but rather for their personal gratification – often unconsciously. This means that you are the one who must learn to listen to your needs, to be firm and assertive, rather than just hope others will guess what your needs are.

When you can say NO without feeling guilty, without fear of hurting someone or losing their love, you will also more easily understand others who refuse what *you* offer: they are not saying they don't love you, they are just listening to their own needs.

If you respect the needs of others, you will also not make an effort to deprive them. I am alluding here especially to people who are very strict about the diets of those close to them – their children, their partner, an aging parent in their care. Have you been involved in that kind of situation? Your intentions are surely good, out of concern for their health or their weight, but this attitude is nevertheless disrespectful. If you show your rigid side like this with those you love, it goes without saying that you treat yourself the same way. This is yet another example of operating in control mode.

Moreover, when you stop trying to influence others, you will notice that others will make less effort to have influence over you. In conclusion, the more you respect the dietary needs of the members of your family, the more you will notice them developing respect for you. By respect, I mean respect in all areas. Remember that diet is only a reflection of what is going on in the other areas of your life.

Avoiding conflicts
during mealtimes

With today's hectic lifestyle, a lot of people unfortunately only see each other at mealtimes. And then, they often spend this precious time arguing, blaming, criticizing, complaining, giving out orders, and so forth. It's the surest way *not* to benefit from your food: swallow it fast, don't bother to taste, don't smell anything, just hope the meal will be over as soon as possible.

If you experience this kind of situation in your life, it can be a good idea to ask the members of your family if they could all agree and promise to discuss only pleasant things during mealtime. Agree on some sort of signal or key word to use as a reminder when, for example, someone starts negative behaviour and forgets their commitment. At first, it will be normal that some people forget, but gradually, you will manage to adopt this new habit, something that will benefit everyone tremendously.

When we criticize or feel criticized or judged while we are ingesting food, it is impossible for our stomach to digest it properly. Why is that? Because when we cannot tolerate or "digest" another person or a situation, it affects the physical digestion of our food. I want to repeat that it is never a food that is difficult to digest, but it is our inner state of indigestion or of criticism that is affecting our stomach. When we eat with love and acceptance and letting go, the body, offering no resistance, does its work quite naturally.

Avoiding distractions during mealtimes

According to statistics, about 75% of people say they eat together as a family. But there is a new phenomenon occurring: people are being distracted. Indeed, the same statistics show that 33% of people say they leave the television on during their meals or use that time to read the newspaper or a favourite book. Today, there are even more distractions that come into play: cordless phones, cell phones, texting, e-mailing... As a result, people are not paying attention to what they eat or to the quantities they are consuming. They are preoccupied with other activities.

Above I mentioned avoiding conflicts during mealtimes. Distractions produce the same effect as conflicts: people become completely disconnected from their family.

If you see yourself reflected in these examples, I recommend that you try an experiment: abstain from distractions for at least three weeks -- so as to give it a chance. Don't you think three weeks represents a relatively short period of time in your life for an experiment that could prove to be truly beneficial for you and your family?

If several of you eat meals together, you may not all agree with this idea, but you can always negotiate. You might take one three-week period to try the experiment with those who are interested and then another three-week period for those who prefer to keep bringing their favourite distraction to the table. You might even decide that each group will take their meals in a different area for the duration of the experiment. These are only suggestions. I am sure that together you can find a solution.

Knowing when you are hungry and when you are no longer hungry

It may be that it is difficult for you to know when you really are hungry, even if you ask yourself all the questions suggested on page... It will be especially hard if you had the habit of eating out of gourmandise – fondness for food – or out of emotion, never giving yourself the chance to get hungry. Remember that it takes a certain amount of time for any new habit to become routine.

Why? Because your body has stopped sending you signals that you were barely listening to anyway. Look at this example of a woman who had the bad habit of losing her temper easily. She wants to become more tolerant and patient because the family atmosphere has become unpleasant and she doesn't want to be feeling guilty about this anymore. But despite her desire to change her attitude, she doesn't manage to achieve this. So she asks her husband to do her a favour and alert her every time she gets angry, by giving her a signal the two of them have agreed on. After several weeks of her husband's co-operation on this, she nevertheless continues to ignore his signals and her outbursts are still just as frequent. How long do you think her husband will continue to help her before he gives up?

If for some time already you have not been paying attention to your body's signals that it is hungry or full, i.e., no longer hungry, it is quite possible that it has ceased all communication, all efforts to send you messages. I have come to realize that for most people, it is even harder to know when they have stopped being hungry than it is to

113

know when they are hungry. Don't get discouraged. With practice and perseverance, we can achieve anything.

That reminds me of the time when, a few years ago, I began to do a set of exercises called The Five Tibetan Rites every morning. When a friend taught me these exercises, I could hardly raise my body from the ground. I could not imagine that one day I would manage to become as flexible as she was. To my great surprise, I succeeded, thanks to perseverance, and I am very proud of it. After many years, these exercises have now become very easy, even as my body ages.

One suggestion I would offer, to help you detect the moment when you are no longer hungry, is to ask yourself, when you are halfway through your meal, whether you are still hungry. Generally speaking, the answer will be yes. So, then, you continue, but stopping at regular intervals to ask yourself the same question. Little by little, you will know when you are no longer hungry. You will be able to recognize your own personal signal. For some people, the food stops tasting good. For others, they just feel "stuffed". For still others, their throat seems to close up. And there are those who can simply tell, without receiving any special clue.

Another accepted fact is that when we drink while eating, it is much harder to tell when we are no longer hungry. The liquid mixed with the ball of food distorts the information conveyed to the body and prevents it from sending the expected signal that it is satisfied. The recommendation, therefore, is to drink either before or after the meal.

If you are someone who has learned that it is wrong to leave food on your plate, that you must ALWAYS eat it

ALL, then it must be very difficult for you to know when you are no longer hungry. According to statistics, at least 54% of people are like you: their plate must be empty before they leave the table. There are even people who cannot help thoroughly cleaning their plate with a piece of bread or who finish what other people leave on their plate, believing that one must NEVER THROW OUT FOOD. They become the family garbage can themselves.

This belief has created a problem that previous generations did not face.

Serving portions in restaurants have become much larger since the sixties and eating out has become more popular. This belief, then, is making people eat larger portions and it is affecting their health and their weight. We can know this by observing how the percentage of obese people increases year after year.

If you wait for a signal telling you that you can't handle one more mouthful, and feel completely stuffed, you will have the unpleasant feeling of having overeaten and at that point it is too late. The real signal that the body is satisfied is given well before this stage. If you encounter this situation, take a few moments to ask yourself when you think it was time to stop. Which part was too much? The answers may be helpful to you in future. The answer might be, *The last five mouthfuls were too much,* or *The second slice of bread dipped in gravy* or perhaps *It was the dessert I could have done without.*

Do not forget, and this is very important, that if you go and feel guilty about this, it will be even harder for your body to digest and eliminate this excess food. Replace this guilt with a consciousness of what the heaviness you feel in your physical body is trying to tell you. It wants to draw attention to the fact that your emotional and mental bodies are currently being overburdened and overtaxed, that you are weighing yourself down with thoughts that are not beneficial to you. They might be fears or grudges... The fastest way to ease this load is to move into genuine love and acceptance of yourself in the midst of whatever is taking place that day.

Then ask your body to kindly eliminate this excess rather than converting it into fat, reminding it that you are trying to learn to listen to it better so as to know when it has had enough. Ask it not to give up on you. Gradually, it will have less work to do, as you grow in your ability to love yourself, which will result in attentive listening to your body's needs. I have noticed that this attitude produces remarkable results. Our body, sensing inner acceptance, listens to us and eliminates what it doesn't need instead of storing it and gaining weight.

Eating without feeling guilty helps your body eliminate this surplus, even when you give it extra work to do. Furthermore, if you feel guilty, the harmful consequences will show up on all levels. However, people who often eat too much or don't eat what they need and still never gain weight risk developing problems with their digestive system.

This feeling of having overeaten often occurs with those who eat out of compulsion, who are trying to fill an inner void caused by a lack of self-love. It is important then to accept ourselves in this situation and to thank our body for helping us to become conscious that it is time to learn to love ourselves more.

Do you sometimes say to yourself: I can't just throw out what's left on my plate, that would be really wasteful or This is just too good, I can't stop even if I know I'm not really hungry anymore or I want to take maximum advantage of all these delectable dishes available while I'm on holiday or at friends. If so, you can see the excuses you are giving yourself for not listening to your body. You have been in the habit of controlling your diet – and trying to control your life – for so long that your ego is frightened by the realization that you now want to start being your own master, that is, you want to listen to the needs of your physical body. It does not believe you'll be able to assume the consequences of that decision and is convinced it will be too hard for you to do without the psychological compensation you've been getting from food. This is why you have to go through the experience, in order to reassure your ego that, yes, you can assume the consequences, without this decision necessarily being too hard on you. What you need to realize above all is that **the suffering associated with consuming foods your body does not need has become greater than the suffering associated with the lack of psychological compensation.**

One method you can use if you find it difficult to leave food on your plate is to imagine that in some unseen way you are able to send these good leftovers to someone in the world who needs them. I am so convinced of each of our intentions being immediately translated by universal energy that at that same instant someone in need will find or will be offered food.

Another question people ask themselves is *Do I need to eat as soon as I feel hungry?* It is true that when we are learning to feel genuine hunger again, we notice it sooner.

117

It is preferable not to wait too long after the first signs of hunger. Why? Because otherwise the body will think that you want to deprive it and will go into prevention mode. It will want to stock up on reserves.

You could compare this situation to when the body calls us to eliminate waste. There is no need to run to the toilet, but it is best to answer the call as soon as possible. People who wait till the last minute are not listening to their body. They are torturing it needlessly – as they torture themselves in their daily lives. If you recognize yourself in the picture I have just described, you must have noticed how insensitive you have become to your body's signals, and it is very likely that you suffer from constipation.

In fact, it is better to eat several times a day than to deprive yourself when you are hungry. It may seem paradoxical to claim that eating this way will result in less weight gain than when you try to control yourself, but it is an established fact. I have noticed, during workshops, that certain women come with a small stash of food, like nuts or nutrition bars, etc. to snack on at intervals during the day. The snacks are not big, but seem to be taken frequently. Yet these women have no weight problem whatsoever. The important thing is to be sure that you received the signal from your body telling you it is hungry. Eating several times a day can of course also turn out to be a dependency or a habit. Only you will be able to tell if this is the case, as long as you are paying attention.

If you are the type of person who stops eating before your body tells you it is satisfied, you're going to feel hungry again quite soon aren't you? It is preferable to nourish your body when it needs it and not to control it by telling yourself you can't eat between meals. You know as well as I do that anyone who applies control in the area of food tends to lose that same control in another area, like shouting for no reason, crying uncontrollably, dramatizing trivial situations, etc.

Eating what you like

But still, you can't always be eating whatever you feel like. I like a lot of fattening things, that are greasy or very salty, that make my skin break out, that are hard to digest... Does that sound like you? I wouldn't be surprised if it did because I have often heard these kinds of comments. This type of thinking is maintained by those who believe that, all the same, it is necessary to restrain oneself and have a certain degree of control because otherwise it would be considered "letting yourself go".

Have you noticed where control has gotten you so far? Over the course of the years, have you stopped feeling guilty whenever you yielded to temptation, when you were unable to restrain yourself? The answer is no, isn't it? I have yet to meet someone who could answer yes to this question. Surely you have realized that the more often you say that you should not do something, or that you should achieve this or that, the more you keep feeling guilty in addition to being unable to achieve what you want. This is no doubt the most vicious circle in the world.

We think that by feeling guilty, the little voice – the ego – in our head will stop repeating to us: *this is not good.* Alas, it is the opposite that happens. What are you supposed to do, then? You will be shocked at what I am going to suggest. Choose a favourite food and eat as much of it as often as you want, even every day. Take the time to warn your body first that you are about to undertake an experiment. Tell it you want to give yourself the right to eat whatever you feel like in order to find out whether a particular food is harmful to your body or not, that is, when you have really felt and experienced the effects for yourself. You don't have to listen to people who claim that a particular food is bad for you without ever having checked out the consequences by trying it for themselves. They are convinced of the theory by virtue of having heard about it and decided to accept as true what others believed to be true.

However, you must follow through all the way with your experiment. I guarantee you that if you can do this without feeling any guilt, you will feel and know within a very short time whether this food is harmful to you or not. In fact, your objective is to come to a decision as to whether to stop or modify your intake of this food, only because it is no longer an intelligent thing to do to hurt yourself, not because it is "bad" to eat it. As soon as you stop a behaviour because a little voice tells you to stop, tells you it's not good, it becomes control, and it isn't you – it isn't your heart – that is deciding, but rather your ego, which likes to perpetuate the idea of good and bad in you.

If you find yourself in a loss-of-control situation and are unable to stop, it is an indication that you are feeling guilty again. If it is just too difficult for you to do this exercise without feeling guilty, try it as an experiment with a different food, reminding yourself that one day you'll come back and try it with a favourite food. No one can do this for you. Only you can succeed in transforming the way you think about the things you like. This is the way to proceed, with one food at a time.

You have nothing to lose by trying this new attitude and adopting this new behaviour because before, even when you tried to control yourself, you kept falling back into a loss of control. Besides, you might have the pleasant surprise of discovering that your belief that a certain food was bad for you, or didn't agree with you, was false and that your body is just fine with it and may even need this food.

One day a woman told me what her mother had told her when she was an adolescent: *If you want to lose weight, it's very simple, just stop eating EVERYTHING you like.* You can imagine the weight problem and the guilt that this woman experienced all her life. As soon as she savoured anything, the little voice in her head reminded her incessantly, like a broken record, that she was going to gain weight. There you have another belief that would prevent you from eating food you enjoy.

Any belief we hold should be kept only if it is beneficial for us to do so. As soon as we realize that something we believe is making our life difficult, preventing us from being well, from being free and listening to our needs, we know that from that moment forward, it is no longer intelligent for us to hold on to that belief. So, **you do not have to ask yourself whether what you believe is true or not, but rather whether the beliefs you hold make you happy or not and bring you the desired results or not.**

Every belief creates new connections in the brain. And the more a belief settles in, the more the connection becomes important. Our ways of thinking, our actions and our reactions are mostly involuntary. Do you realize how often you act without thinking, without reflecting? It is true that at times we can be listening to our needs and still be spontaneous, but we are nevertheless more inclined to listen to our ego than to our heart. We may think we are the ones directing our lives but, actually, we are not. Do you aspire to one day being master of your actions and reactions, your thoughts and decisions?

To get there, you'll need to accept that, for now, it won't always be you that's directing your life. Next, you take the decision that, starting now, you want to develop new habits that will benefit you.

It takes at least three months to create a new habit or introduce a different way of acting or thinking. This allows the brain the time it needs to create a new connection and adjust to new data, and delete, so to speak, the former automatic reflex. Giving ourselves more than one choice in any given situation helps us to develop our ability to discern and not to behave like robots.

Suppose you are the type of person who, each time they pass a dish of candy, cannot help but scoop up a handful – at a restaurant, in a waiting room, at your grandmother's place, or at a supermarket promotion stand… Until now, you have created the automatic reaction of taking a handful of candies, popping some into your mouth and putting some in your pocket or purse "just in case".

To begin the shift, you decide to take as much as you want, choosing to believe that this behaviour is no longer "bad". Afterwards, you find other ways to act in this same situation. Sometimes you don't take any, sometimes you take just one, or you take several and eat them all. At other times you eat one and offer the rest to someone else and, finally, you could perhaps decide to throw them in the garbage while visualizing that you are sending sugar to someone who really needs it, somewhere in the world. Through this practice, you will learn that there are many ways to handle the identical situation and that you can always master it.

If the word *cheat* is part of your vocabulary or maybe you think about it often, it would be a good idea to transform this habit. As soon as the word "cheat" comes to mind, you have just learned that you feel guilty. It's the beginning of another vicious circle. Since you feel guilty about having cheated, it is almost guaranteed that you will continue to eat more of this food to punish yourself more, because you hate yourself when you act this way. And sometimes people accuse themselves of "cheating" when their body really needed that food. When they blame themselves, they eat more of it than necessary.

After you have cheated, you promise yourself not to start again, believing that this is the way to stop your craving. However, it's actually the opposite inclination that is being created. The more you tell yourself that you will not start again, the more you do start again. This is why there is so much guilt in the world. We think that by feeling very guilty, we will not start again and that it is an indication that we are a good person. We judge people who do not feel guilty as being indifferent.

The only way to transform behaviour is through acceptance. That is to say, to give oneself the right to have limits instead of accusing or lecturing oneself and prompting unrealistic promises. Acceptance is a letting-go. **The more you let go, the more things change. The more you want to control things, the less they change.**

Eating what you don't like

I have just raised the fact that we often like and eat things that we know or believe our body doesn't need. It also happens that we eat things we do not like. Afterwards, we ask ourselves why we chose to consume it regardless.

This sort of thing happens mostly when we want to reward ourselves the way Mom or someone in her place did. Parents often reward their children with food without checking if it is something they like: for example, a piece of carrot cake or cheese cake, while the child might not care for this dessert.

Now, since the child perceives they are receiving a reward in the form of this food, they make an effort to eat it because they feel loved, accepted, acknowledged by their mom. They eat it, not because it tastes good and they like it, but rather for the psychological pleasure associated with this food.

If, when you make your daily journal entries, you become conscious of this fact, take the time to thank yourself for having come to this new awareness and resolve that you can reward yourself in a different way in future. You don't need rewards or approval from Mom anymore. It is indeed your approval that counts from now on and that's going to make all the difference for you.

And then there are those who continue to eat this food despite having noticed that they dislike it. It might be in a restaurant or a situation where someone has offered them this food. They are the type of person who, to their own detriment, is afraid of offending or upsetting others.

If you see yourself in this example, when you are filling out your journal, you should know that you are doing the same thing in the other areas of your life. In the Link column, find the situation where you had difficulty expressing your unhappiness or saying you didn't like something, out of fear of upsetting or hurting the other person. Then you will become aware of a new situation in which you need to learn to love yourself more. It's your fear that is influencing you to give your body something you do not need and furthermore, that your taste buds don't even like. When you express your need in future, you will discover that most of the time, it doesn't hurt or bother others in the least. Noticing this will enable you succeed in letting go of your fear.

Food allergies and food intolerances

There is a phenomenon occurring in several countries these days that may prove to be very revealing for many people. I am talking about the considerable increase in food allergies and food intolerances. It is a phenomenon that often develops at an early age and can continue for a long time, even an entire lifetime. Other times it shows up in adulthood.

A food allergy generates more harmful – sometimes even dangerous – consequences than a food intolerance. The difference between the two conditions can be explained this way: A **food allergy** consists of a sensitivity provoked by a reaction of the immune system to a particular protein found in a food. This chain reaction is therefore responsible for symptoms such as serious breathing problems and/or skin problems.

A **food intolerance** consists of a food sensitivity that does not involve a reaction by the individual's immune system. Rather, it is liable to show up in the gastro-intestinal system and is usually caused by an inability to digest or absorb certain foods or food elements.

The words used to describe these two conditions speak for themselves. Allergy... sensitivity... reaction... intolerance... problems... inability to digest.

People who decide to remove a certain food from their diet, thinking that their body is refusing to digest it, would benefit greatly from using this phenomenon as a tool to get to know themselves better. In reality it is not the food that is hard to digest, it is another person.

If this applies to you, take the time to ask, *What does this food represent for me?* or *What does it make me think of?* You may end up discovering major emotions that have been repressed in you waiting impatiently to be discovered so that you may liberate yourself from them.

For example, I know a woman who's body couldn't tolerate cucumbers. Forty years later, she was able to make the connection between cucumber and the sexual abuse she had suffered when she was young. The cucumber brought back to her mind the distressing image of the acts her father had subjected her to. Once she was able to truly forgive him, she was able to eat cucumbers again without a problem.

In my own case, any soup that contained tomato got stuck in my throat. I would run to the toilet to throw it up each time I tried again to see if I could tolerate it. My mother, who could not understand the cause of my adverse reaction, insisted I try again from time to time. One day, I finally realized what this kind of soup reminded me of. It was the nuns who made me eat it several times a week, while I was living in a convent boarding school where I had been placed at the age of five. To me, their soup tasted like dish detergent. I had indigestion and cried every time they forced me to eat it. Years later, I had to put myself through a process of forgiving and accepting these nuns.

All forms of food allergies can be associated with an incident that awakened one of the childhood wounds. This phenomenon shows up particularly in hypersensitive people, those who let themselves be easily affected by others. They often react swiftly and show intolerance. That is why these people are quick to criticize, whether they express it or not. They have trouble "digesting" those toward whom they feel intolerant. If you are allergic to another person, it means you cannot do without them: you seek their presence while at the same time you cannot stand them and criticize them openly.

I suggest that those who have been suffering from an allergy from the time they were very young try doing some decoding. You might think that a one-year-old could not be allergic to another person. Not so. Even from birth, quite unconsciously, our wounds play a role and are activated by members of our family and, consequently, our emotions come into play. It is too easy to believe that our body is reacting just because it does not like a certain food or because its system is refusing it. We need to remember that every physical reaction is symbolic of a psychological reaction.

We know if we don't like a food as soon as we taste it and chew it. So we should then choose not to eat any more of it out of love for ourselves. If you have a reaction after ingesting a spoiled food, this is showing up to draw your attention to the fact that you should have noticed it immediately as soon as you tasted the first mouthful. If you ate all of it in spite of this, it is a sign that you do the same thing in your life. You allow yourself to be influenced by thoughts or people that are trying to poison your life at this time.

As you can observe, there is always a connection to be found between what is happening on the physical level and on the other levels. Nothing is left to chance. Once this fact is well understood and accepted, it is much easier afterwards to discover unconscious aspects of yourself. In the last chapter, we will look at how to manage these emotions through your food habits.

Fear of being hungry

Are you among those who think they have to have three big meals a day to make sure they won't get hungry between meals? Or might you be the kind of person who very often brings food with you when you leave the house because you're afraid you might get hungry? I know a lot of people who claim to feel weak when they are hungry. It is much more the fear of feeling a weakness that is at issue here. That fear can be strong enough to provoke a feeling of lack of energy even though it is very rare for a person not to have enough reserve energy to take them to the next meal. This type of weakness would normally be experienced only when you are severely lacking in nourishment (for example, if you are anorexic) or seriously lacking in an important nutrient. So, here is another opportunity to let go of a fear.

It is true that I mentioned above that on certain days our body prefers several small meals and that on other days one or two meals will prove sufficient. The ideal attitude to adopt is to claim the right to eat in any pattern, that you are not accountable to anyone in this regard and that it is only you who will have to assume the consequences of your decisions.

Realizing that you have the right to eat as often as you wish, it will be easier for you not to feel obliged to consume large meals. Because you know that, should you feel hungry later, you can always take a little something.

I suggest that at first you continue carrying a snack with you. On the other hand, it is important that you choose that "something" wisely. Hard candies or small cookies are certainly not a very healthy way of assuaging your hunger. It would be better to get yourself some foods that offer a good source of energy, like natural almonds, for instance.

Gradually, you will learn that this type of hunger is not serious. You won't be needing to nibble all the time out of fear of feeling unwell if you get too hungry. However, don't forget to remind your body not to worry and that as soon as you can, you will give it nourishment. Your intention is not to put it on a diet or to make it think famine has arrived or is coming.

A varied diet

I have noticed over the years that most people get used to a certain kind of diet and do not think of experimenting with more recent varieties. If this is you, it is very likely that it is also difficult for you to say yes to new situations that present themselves in your life, especially those that are outside your control.

Having the courage to try at least one new food each week may bring very surprising results for you. Are you ready to open yourself to some new life experiences, that will help sharpen your discernment? Then why not start with the area of food? Not only will your body be happy about this initiative, but there will be an additional benefit: it will develop your taste buds.

It is possible that some people will be reluctant to taste new foods because when they were young, any new foods they were offered were poorly prepared or of poor quality. But this wouldn't be the case today because now you are free to choose the quality of the food you want to try out.

The more you try new ingredients or new foods, being sure to do so at a time when you are hungry and chewing the food well, the more you will be able to tell immediately whether your body likes this choice. If you're not sure, there's nothing to stop you from coming back to it later.

Eating naturally

It is more and more difficult to get our nourishment from natural foods because we are consuming increasing quantities of chemicals – most of the time without even realizing it. It is filling our body with toxins in addition to everything we breathe and what our body has to absorb in spite of any efforts we make to the contrary. This pheno-menon has accelerated sharply since the Second World

War, following the major changes that came about in the industrialized countries. Now, even children who are accustomed to eating naturally from the time they are born start finding it hard to do so when they come to adolescence. Junk food becomes hard to resist.

Agriculture has been completely transformed because of the huge quantities of pesticides. Animal husbandry is no longer done in a natural way and as a result, transfers toxins to us that our body does not need. For instance, animals are fed fatty acids that are very rich in Omega-6 and low in Omega-3. Yet it is the latter that are essential to the human body, as it cannot manufacture it. Animals (the ones I call contented animals) that feed naturally produce equal amounts of Omega 6 and Omega 3.

This means that when we eat the meat of these contented animals, or their animal products like milk and eggs, we are accessing a more harmonious diet. However, when we eat the meat of animals raised in the non-traditional – "normal" rather than natural – way, the balance in our body is affected. We stuff our body with products that foul up our system. Many researchers have come to the conclusion that these fatty acids rich in Omega-6, that we find not only in meat, but also in oils, is the main cause – scientifically speaking – of the great plague of obesity that the industrialized countries suffer from increasingly.

This is reason enough to choose the most natural foods possible. There are good books on this topic as well as a vast, ever growing selection of shops and markets where these foods are sold. This is not an invitation to become a vegetarian. Indeed, "natural" does not necessarily mean "vegetarian". If your body asks you for meat, milk and eggs, providing it with organic products does make a big difference. Instead of taking my word for it, why don't you experiment? If you eat meat from animals raised and fed naturally for at least three months, observe the difference it makes on your attitude and behaviour, comparing the effects obtained when you eat products that come from animals that live in fear, anger, rage – in response to the harsh treatment inflicted by some producers – and that have been subjected to what goes on in the slaughterhouse.

To eat natural and organic food is first of all an act of love toward yourself. As we know we cannot dissociate our three 'bodies', our life in general will be affected if we eat this way. If you make a decision to eat more naturally starting now, you will discover that it will be easier for you to be balanced emotionally and mentally, that you will be able to live freely, according to your own nature, in accordance with what you are now and what you want to be.

Even with all the determination in the world to live in a natural environment, it is impossible today not to be exposed to chemical products. We are subjected to them constantly, without our knowledge. This is why it is so important that we do our part as frequently as we can, to help our body. Every time you give your body food that is not natural, your system is thereby weakened. You realize then that you likewise have ways of thinking and beliefs that are weakening you generally.

Physical exercise to detoxify the body

One highly recommended way of detoxifying your body is physical exercise. Even if you make the decision to eat naturally and organically, all these toxins that have accumulated in your body need to be eliminated.

Stress, even psychological stress, affects our physical body in a major way by contributing to the buildup of toxins. All stress is fear-related. As soon as we are afraid, the suprarenal glands produce adrenalin, which has the property of seeking in the tissues and organs the energy needed to handle this fear. Everything follows from that point: the heart beats faster, our breathing accelerates, our blood pressure rises, etc. Since the fear is not real, that is to say, our life is not in any real danger – and the fear is therefore based on something imaginary –, this energy does not get used physically in an act of defense and remains stuck in our body, thus affecting our entire system.

Adopting a pattern of regular physical activity – at least four or five times a week – is a way of helping your body to get rid of those extra toxins. Besides, you will be meeting one of the body's principal needs. So, by engaging in physical exercise, you not only assist your body in the detoxifying process, but you get your body accustomed to listening to an important need, especially as physical activity is an excellent way to unwind and relax. To come home and crash in front of the television, after sitting all day at work, is very unnatural. Your body cries HELP.

I know that the decision to get up earlier in the morning or to get yourself out after an exhausting day of work, to go for a walk or a bike ride or do some kind of sport, is not always easy. On the other hand, the most difficult part is only that minute that it takes to make the decision. Once we are well into the activity, we are proud of our decision. We can feel how happy our body is too.

If you are the type who has trouble disciplining yourself and you soon forget how geared up you were, then, instead of being hard on yourself about this, just give yourself the time you need to let this habit take root. Very often, if people give up along the way, it is because they ask too much of themselves at the beginning. You can start with one day a week for a month and gradually increase to two days a week every month. That way it won't be so drastic and you will feel more encouraged.

It is also recommended that you try different forms of physical exercise, whether it be physical yoga or the use of fitness equipment, until you find out what you are most comfortable with. Even varying the postures or selecting different equipment is a good idea, since each exercise involves a different set of muscles. It is commonly accepted, however, that walking remains the exercise par excellence, as it brings into play almost all the body's muscles and at the same time provides a massage of your internal organs. The walking should be done, however, at a fairly brisk pace, with hands free and arms allowed to swing. As well, if you take the time to be conscious of your breathing in and your breathing out, you are getting an added benefit from your activity. In fact, the air you breathe contains a subtle form of energy called *prana*, which consists of a natural food that the physical body and the subtle – emotional and mental – bodies need. This *prana* can even help reduce hunger, without adding calories!

We now know that physical activity provokes the secretion of certain hormones in the brain, called endorphins. These hormones have properties comparable to those of morphine. They are relaxing and therefore an excellent tool for counteracting fears and stress. They are also stimulating and energizing.

Another benefit of exercise is the intimate communion between you and your body that results from the attention it gets from you. Your body will be much more willing to co-operate with you, for example, in letting you know clearly and precisely when you really are hungry, what you need when you are hungry and the point when your hunger has been satisfied.

If there are times you find it impossible to exercise or to do any physical activity and if, moreover, on that particular day, you feel a lot of tension or stress, you might want to use the following method. Find a spot – it could be in a corner of your house – where you can scream, punch a pillow, cry as much as you want. Give yourself about ten minutes to do this and, after that, say in a firm and strong voice, THAT'S ENOUGH. It will subsequently be easier for you to be introspective and discover the fears you have in yourself – and for yourself – that have been the cause of so much stress. As you can see, there are several ways to let go of a great many useless things in our life.

Breathing

Taking the time to breathe deeply is another important factor that helps us be able to let go. Have you noticed that while you are reading this book you are not really conscious of your breathing? You are no doubt letting air into your lungs through an involuntary reflex. This phenomenon takes place almost all day. We are so involved in our activities that we forget about this vital function. Even if breathing is a totally autonomous function of the body, it is also easily controlled by the will. Therefore it is good to utilize any moments where it is feasible to take the time to breathe in and out deeply.

When we talk about breathing deeply, it is not just a matter of inhaling long breaths as this could actually cause hyperventilation. A few long inhalations and exhalations are suggested only to help us relax. Being conscious of your breathing means observing the air that enters your lungs, following its movement – not forcing it – until you feel your sides expand. You know at that point that the air has filled your lungs correctly. Afterwards you feel your sides contracting as the air is expelled.

This healthful type of breathing brings many benefits. It helps you be calmer, be in closer contact with your body, and develop a greater aptitude for listening to your body. It is impossible to really tune in to your inner self if your breathing is always shallow. Train yourself to become conscious of your breathing as often as possible... when driving your car, while waiting in line at the bank or supermarket... and gradually, you will learn greater mastery of your breathing.

Furthermore, when you are eating, if you inhale and exhale consciously, at least once between mouthfuls, it will help you identify the moment when you are no longer hungry. When you fill in your daily journal at the end of each day, why not add how many times you were aware of your breathing?

Light, energy and gratitude

Every time you ingest food, it is a good idea to visualize this food bathed in light. This will help you to energize everything you eat. In fact, you do not need to believe in this statement. When I started to practice this new habit, I had no idea of its benefits. So, I said to myself, *What do I have to lose?* When you learn about something that is unlikely to do you any harm and stands a good chance of doing you some good, why not go with it? I recognize that I have a lot more energy than the average person my age and I attribute this, in large part, to all these good habits that I acquired over the years.

I use this method especially when I am in a restaurant where I am eating foods that are not that natural, in circumstances where I have no control over their quality. I surround my food with light while asking my body to absorb only what is good of what I eat and to eliminate as quickly as possible what is not beneficial for me.

Also in this regard, giving thanks to all those who have contributed to the production or creation of the food – from planting the seed through to preparing the dish – adds another energizing element: all gratitude energizes both the one thanked and the one who is thankful.

If you are thinking you'll never be able to remember all the above suggestions every time you take food, I understand your apprehension. It takes practice for something to become a habit. Every good habit can only create amazing consequences for you. It's another great sign of self-love. **Remember that you receive love from others in the same degree as you love yourself.**

Start by developing just one habit at a time. When the first one is well rooted and has become a part of you, then you start on the next one. It's like learning to drive a car. At first, a lot of effort is required to think of everything, but gradually, it becomes easier. You will realize when you come down to it that this reflex only takes a few seconds at each meal. You could use a short personal code to help you remember. For instance, place the word LOVE or LIGHT in a prominent place in your kitchen. Any strategies that are liable to help you with this goal are valuable.

Knowing if it is beneficial for you

At times, you may have a sudden craving for a food that, in your belief system, would be categorized as "not good for you". When that happens, do you know how to recognize whether your desire represents a need your body has? There is only one way to tell. Delay your response to this craving for awhile, busy yourself with something else and if the craving slips from your mind, it is an indication that it was nothing more than a passing desire, not a need. On the other hand, if your taste for this food is still present a few hours later, please, do yourself a favor and enjoy it with love.

I only recommend taking this approach when you feel like having a food considered "bad for you", since I want to remind you that if you really are hungry, it is better to eat right away.

Even if your body does not really need it, this food will benefit you in ways beyond the physical. It is probably the only means you know to reward yourself at that moment.

By accepting this inability to reward yourself in a different way at that moment, you will learn a new way much faster. Otherwise, if you do not satisfy this persistent desire and you restrain yourself, you know that you will lose control again at some point anyway.

If you are among those who seek to satisfy all their slightest little cravings and whims instantly, without checking to see if it is really necessary, in the various areas of your life other than food, then you must also want to satisfy your desire for food instantly. This kind of behaviour is often influenced by something missing in your emotional life.

How can you develop greater discernment to help you distinguish between food that is beneficial for you and food that is not? Give yourself the right to try everything, to eat and drink whatever appeals to you, being aware all the while of what is going on in you and especially paying no attention to what others tell you. No one in the world can really know what is good for another person. Something can be very good for one person and bad for another.

An excellent method that lets you know whether what you are preparing to eat is beneficial for your body – i.e., whether your body really needs it – is to chew the first mouthful really well, chew it until it becomes completely liquid. Sometimes I really feel like having something and then, right after the first mouthful that I've chewed, the food becomes acid in my mouth or leaves an unpleasant taste. I know then that the desire for that food does not correspond to a genuine need. It is easier after that to make the connection between this false desire and what is hiding behind it.

Let me share a personal example to illustrate this point. One day while I was at home in the late afternoon, following an intense period of writing and a few phone calls, I had a strong craving for potato chips. Almost immediately after the first mouthful, an acid taste filled my mouth. Why then did I feel that need? The answer came to me within a fraction of a second. I had experienced a lot of impatience during the phone calls. I kept getting automated messages offering me various options, none of which corresponded to what I was looking for. After the last call and several waiting periods with the same marketing message and the same voice asking the caller to be patient, I learned I would be transferred and for some reason or another, I would have to start this long litany of messages all over again. In short, having run out of patience, I basically slammed the receiver down. I was fed up. I then found myself in the kitchen.

Those chips, for which I had an irresistible desire and that I thought I really needed, were playing the role of appeasing my anger. At that moment, I felt an immediate need to bite into something in order to compensate for not having shown toward those representatives the biting attitude I had felt. I had restrained myself with them, knowing they had little to say about the matter, that it was their company that made those policies. I also restrained myself because I would have felt guilty about expressing my anger while knowing that these people who work in the customer service department are usually very friendly and patient. It is difficult to be severe and impatient with them without feeling guilty afterwards. That was the source of my desire to compensate by having something dry and crusty that I didn't need.

The times when I eat these kinds of chips and they taste good are the times when I allow myself to use them as a reward, without any sense of guilt. A reminder that listening to your body does not mean that you ALWAYS give our body what it needs. Listening to your body and listening to your needs are two different things. **Listening to our body, means using our physical body (and in this case, using the way we eat) to become conscious of what is going on inside us. To listen to our needs is to know what our three bodies (physical, emotional and mental) really need.**

Then, if we have feelings of anger, impatience, sadness, boredom, or aggressivity, for example, we will be able to tell how well we accept these emotions by observing whether we are able to choose foods likely to help us compensate for these feelings without guilt.

Let's take the instance of a woman who feels angry toward a colleague at work. She gets home and finds she just wants to let loose somehow and before she knows it, she's got the ice cream container out. While she's eating some, if she is aware that she doesn't really need it, but is using this way to let go, she will be able to stop before she has stuffed herself by finishing up all the ice cream. She has given herself the right to behave this way for now. If she, furthermore, acknowledges to her body that she knows it has no need of this food and asks it to indulge her and eliminate what it doesn't need as quickly as possible, there will be no harmful effect. Thanking her body in advance for the extra work she is imposing on it shows she has a loving rather than a guilty attitude.

I must warn you on the other hand that it is not always easy to know if you are really accepting yourself. So, you can make yourself believe you accept yourself even when it isn't really true. As is the case for most people, there are several stages to go through before reaching self-acceptance.

- ♦ The first stage generally consists of self-deprivation and self-control, based on how unacceptable we find a particular behaviour.

- ♦ Next, we engage in the behaviour but feel guilty afterwards.

- ♦ The third stage is to make ourselves believe we accept our behaviour by denying our feelings of guilt.

- ♦ And finally, we reach the point of giving ourselves the right.

It is only after this last stage that we are able to master the situation. Note that I am saying *master* and not *control*. We know we have mastery when we choose to act a certain way voluntarily, and are prepared to take the consequences. One way to really know if we accept ourselves is to observe the attitude others have toward us. If they blame us and judge us, it is an indication that we still feel guilty.

Those who do not manage to reach the point of self-acceptance may end up suffering from bulimia, anorexia or hyperphasia. Indeed, there has been a marked increase in these diet-related conditions, particularly in the industrialized countries. What is the connection between these more serious, sometimes extremely serious, problems and what is happening on the psychological level? If you suffer from these problems, here is what you can learn about yourself...

Bulimia

The bulimic person constantly experiences an uncontrollable sensation of hunger. This leads them to eat frantically and to excess. Afterwards, they induce vomiting, take a laxative or do some extreme exercising in order to maintain their weight. Statistics tell us this problem occurs in nine times as many women as men.

I mentioned at the beginning of this book that there is a direct connection between the way we eat and the relationship we had with our mother or the person who had the role of mother for us during our childhood. If you suffer from bulimia, your body is telling you that a part of you misses your mother deeply, to the point where you would like to gobble her up to integrate her into your life. Then you reject her when you make yourself vomit. You experience great inner contradiction. It has probably been this way since you were very young. Through a bulimia problem, you can uncover situations of rejection and abandonment touching both you and your mother. A part of you wants to accept your mother as she is – that's your heart talking – and another part of you wants to reject her – that's your ego, the suffering part, taking over. That's how you behave toward the women in your life, as well as toward yourself, if you are a female. You want to accept them at the same time as you seek to reject them. You find that you are continually in conflict with yourself. When you want to accept your mother, you are afraid because you don't know how to do it and you fear the consequences. So you swing back to rejecting her. Then, in the rejection phase, you do not feel well either. You can see that it just becomes a vicious circle.

Whatever the reasons why you find it difficult to accept your mother, your bulimia problem is an urgent message that it is high time to make your peace with her, to accept her as she is. Since this problem entails a loss of control, try to find the link with the control your mother had over you or the control you would have liked to have over her. It's as if you wanted to control her and at the same time destroy her.

If you are still experiencing this problem, your mother and the women who remind you of your mother are giving you the gift of awakening your suffering – which is what is making you bulimic. The frustration you encounter in your relationships with women is often what triggers an episode of bulimia. It becomes an automatic reaction and when you realize it, it is too late. Instead of feeling guilty, tell yourself that you are a victim of this bulimia for now and that gradually, you will learn to be your own master, that it is not within your capacity to resolve this problem immediately. As soon as you take the decision to make peace with your mother, the problem will diminish. It is a matter of deciding and then acting on your decision.

Making peace with your mother means having compassion for her. Know that she went through the same thing with her mother, that she suffered just as much as you. Talking to her about your feelings could assuredly help both of you. When I say have compassion, I am not talking about agreeing with everything you went through with her, but just putting yourself in her shoes and feeling that she has the same wounds as you do and that you need to forgive each other for having engaged in a behaviour of rejection toward each other. You will find more details on the subject of forgiveness in the next chapter. Rejecting another person does not necessarily make you a mean person. It is simply that you are suffering and do not know how else to handle the situation at that moment. You are so afraid of rejecting someone that it is exactly what you end up doing. You remember, don't you, that the more we promise ourselves not to start again, the more we do start again.

Hyperphasia

Hyperphasia presents like bulimia except that the subject does not use any method to reject the large quantity of food that has just been ingested. It is characterized, rather, by permanent snacking or a far above average intake of food. This person suffers, therefore, from being overweight, in contrast to those who are bulimic or anorexic and obsessed by the fear of gaining weight.

If you recognize yourself in the above description, it means that you want to *gobble up* your mother constantly: you never get enough of her. You no doubt have a very close bond with her. On the other hand, the emotional food you receive from your mother is not what you are looking for or expect from her. You often feel dissatisfied. Part of you would like to be less dependent on your mother and another part of you cannot do without her. This attitude is unconscious most of the time because you refuse to feel the suffering you experience with her. Is it possible that you are filling up your body in order to better feel what you experience with your mother? Is it also possible that you are destroying yourself by eating this way because you feel guilty about the mental accusations you make about your mother? Your present way of eating is there to help you become aware of what you experience with your mother.

I knew a man who could eat a huge quantity of food in the space of just a few minutes. I had the opportunity to observe him on a number of occasions when I was at his home, without his realizing that I could see him from a distance. If I hadn't seen that with my own eyes, I would have believed him when he stated he was very hungry as he sat down at the table half an hour later. At the meal, he consumed a good-size serving as usual. He didn't seem to have the slightest recollection of his clandestine eating in the corner of his kitchen. Consequently, this man has always had an obesity problem.

Around the time I was developing my interest in behavioural problems relating to food, I asked him several questions about his relationship with his mother. He shared with me the fact that he had always been ashamed of his mother and that one day he told himself he no longer had anything in common with her and decided to cut all ties with her. He also confided to me that when she died, he did not feel anything and that he has never mourned her or missed her. I understood then how much he was locked inside his denial regarding his mom. Especially when I learned that he did not understand why she used to tell other members of the family that he had always been her favourite and that she missed him a lot. Having always controlled himself in order to avoid feeling his legitimate need of his mother and the guilt for having completely cut himself off from her, he lost his control when it came to food. There was absolutely no way he wanted to admit he needed his mom.

If you find that you are suffering from hyperphasia, I suggest to you also that you make your peace with your mother and with yourself, as explained in the segment on bulimia and in the last chapter.

Anorexia

In the world of medicine, anorexia is defined in two ways. There is **functional anorexia**, which is the loss of appetite. And then there is **mental anorexia**, which is a psychic problem that translates specifically into significant weight loss. The latter is related to *voluntarily* determined dietary restriction, even if the causes of these self-inflicted deprivations remain unconscious for those suffering from them. In summary, with mental anorexia, the patient fights hunger, while in the case of functional anorexia, they have lost their appetite.

If you are suffering from **mental anorexia**, it is a sign that you completely reject your mother. Again, statistics show there is only one man for every nine women affected by this condition.

If you are a man, your mother was your first model of the feminine principle. By rejecting your mother, you are also rejecting the feminine principle in you. You must also be inclined to reject women in general without knowing exactly why.

If you are a woman, you are rejecting the mother and the woman in you, as well as your femininity. If you have children, you must certainly fear being or becoming the same kind of mom your mother was and, in doing everything possible to assume the role of the perfect mom, you rarely agree with yourself. It is very likely that you often question your behaviour as a woman or as a mother.

Presenting a skinny body that is not very sexually appealing might seem – unconsciously – like a good idea to you as a way of rejecting the fact of becoming a woman.

This is why the problem of anorexia is for the most part triggered in adolescents when they enter puberty.

The issue seems less serious when it is **functional anorexia**, because it is a temporary condition. It is usually triggered by a traumatic experience, a shock, or a major illness. This type of rejection of the feminine is therefore not permanent. The effects of mental anorexia are, for its part, much more harmful. Some people even die from it.

Seeking unrealistic perfection is another very common characteristic of anorexic individuals. It is urgent for you to realize what a fantastic person you are and for you to learn to allow yourself pleasure rather than denying yourself all enjoyment related to food or sex. Rejecting yourself that strongly is indicative of constant guilt feelings with respect to what you are and what you do. You ask far too much of yourself and your expectations are very unrealistic.

If you think that cutting yourself off like that from physical pleasure is going to help you pay the price of your guilt, I regret to have to inform you that your belief is mistaken. The more you seek to punish yourself, the more your guilt will grow. So, instead of feeling guilty about what you are, why not take the attitude that whatever you decide you want to be in life, it is you that will be assuming the consequences. Accept the fact, as well, that **there are no mistakes in life, there are only experiences that help us develop our powers of discernment.**

So, you can decide to be what you wish and do what you wish and follow through on that decision without being obliged to explain or justify it to anyone. And especially you can decide to allow yourself to have more pleasure in your life. It is by assuming the consequences of your choices and decisions that you will become more conscious of what is intelligent and beneficial for you.

That's the main reason why anyone should decide to transform some aspect of themselves. They can thus discover what is the more intelligent option for them. They should not try to change because a little voice inside is telling them something is wrong, making them feel guilty about the way they are. They should rather listen to the voice of their heart, begging them to accept themselves. That's the voice that is right. By accepting themselves, they will find it easier to accept their mother who also suffered rejection, just as they did.

Obsessive behaviour

The above three food-related behavioral problems have to do with obsession. However, food-related obsessive behavior is not limited to those three types.

For instance, are you someone who might plan their menu several days in advance, taking great care to avoid certain products that are considered "bad" for you? Or do you deprive yourself of several foods that you like in order to be sure you are always eating a healthy diet? Are you looking for total perfection in the way you eat to the point where it isolates you more and more from your social life and your family? Those are all obsessive behaviours.

Generally, these behaviours are used to try to calm a deep anxiety. That's why this type of person must compensate with food, either by controlling themselves or by losing control. It's as if at the moment when this anxiety strikes them, it's the only strategy they can use, believing they are diminishing their anxiety this way. But it becomes a vicious circle because the means used to diminish their anxiety causes them another form of anxiety: they feel powerless to slow down this obsessive behaviour.

It has been noted by psychoanalysts – and I have been able to verify this many times – a large percentage of people dealing with behavioural problems around food experienced sexual abuse during childhood or adolescence. When we speak of sexual abuse, we are not necessarily talking about sexual acts. Many children and adolescents may feel abused in their body simply through insinuating looks or words on the part of adults who played the role of parents. Fear of sexual abuse can likewise cause as much damage as abuse itself. For instance, the young girl who sees her father commit incest with her big sister may be traumatized by this, even if her father never touches her personally.

We often link sexual appetite with the appetite for food. A woman may promise herself to keep her sex drive in check and experience a loss of control in the area of food as a result. Moreover, having a very large body, or a very skinny body, makes her believe she will be less desirable and therefore less likely to attract, or find herself in, abusive situations.

I came to realize over my twenty-seven years of teaching, after I had met numerous people who demonstrated an obsessive personality type, that these people have an inferiority complex as big as their guilt complex. As they are passive by nature, these feelings are repressed and intensified without their realizing it. As a consequence, they develop great bitterness and often even hatred toward one of

150

their parents or a person who filled that role. Hatred develops when we repress or deny the pain we experience.

How does this bitterness lead to an obsessive personality? This type of person represses their rancour so much – even denying it completely – that it continues to grow in them like an elemental substance and starts taking up more and more room in the emotional and mental bodies. To deny their bitterness demands increased mental effort and one's constant attention so that it becomes a fixation. This is how they develop their obsessive personality. The stronger the bitterness or hatred, the bigger the obsession becomes.

I have also had the pleasure of noting the great difference in attitude and behaviour in these people after they have truly forgiven the other person and themselves. I cannot help but speak about forgiveness in all the books I write, in all the Listen To Your Body workshops, as well as in all my lectures. I have so often seen miracles happen following forgiveness, that I know without a doubt that it is the very best way to achieve healing, whether of the physical, emotional or mental sort. And that's why I'm going to talk more about it in the next chapter.

Chapter Seven

Loving and accepting yourself, whatever your choices

I always come back to true love in my books, my workshops and my lectures. Why? Because we all need to hear it repeated, over and over and over again. Even if I have been teaching it for twenty-seven years already, I am still as happy as ever to talk about it as much as ever, because it reminds me of the supreme importance of living "in love".

We know we accept ourselves and truly love ourselves when we do not judge in any way our choice of inner attitude and our choice of behaviours. As you have been able to conclude from the earlier chapters, you have certain different behaviours depending on which wounds are activated. This also applies to the way you eat, especially when you do not listen to your needs.

Accepting yourself, in this context, means you give yourself the right, or authorize yourself, to do what you observe yourself doing in the moment, that is, not behaving in accordance with what you want to be – because of one of your wounds. Consequently, you are not truly what you want to be but you are, rather, what you do not want to be. I suggest to you to copy out the following sentence and to place it in a prominent place in your kitchen, if you want to apply this notion of acceptance with respect to food.

I cannot become what I want to be until I have accepted that I am what I do not want to be.

I have written an entire book on the subject of acceptance because there is such strong resistance when it comes to applying this notion. It is always our ego that is at the root of this resistance. Did you know that **the ego does everything in its power to keep us in the past, in order to justify its existence? It wants us to *futurize* – live in the future – in order to ensure its survival**. Therefore, you know immediately that if you are not living in your present moment, it is your ego that is directing you and consequently, you are not listening to your needs.

What is more, as soon as you feel unwell in some way, experience some kind of dissatisfaction, it is a sign that one of your wounds has just been activated, by a situation or a person or by one of your thoughts and again, it is your ego taking over. You are no longer yourself at that moment.

Let us take a look together at how you could learn to accept yourself, according to your different wounds, participating at the same time in healing them, which means that it is you who will be directing your life. Is it not marvelous to be able to use your way of eating to heal your wounds, helping not only your physical body, but also your emotional and mental bodies? This final chapter offers a synthesis of the principal stages of that healing process.

Discovering your wounds

First of all, I suggest that you place your daily journal sheets with the *aide-mémoire* or reminder at the end of this book.

After completing your diet data for the day, note closely the moments when you did not listen to your body. Then take a few moments to check with which wound(s) this way of eating is likely to be linked, referring to Chapter Two. If you are able to do this analysis every day, it will be easier for you to remedy a situation quickly. Otherwise, it is possible you will become aware that the same dietary behaviour – related to an unconscious unpleasant situation – has been repeated for several days and persists. As soon as you realize this, check which control attitude you have developed because of this activated wound, as described in the first chapter. Because of what you have noted in your journal, you are becoming conscious of those moments when it was no longer you that was directing your life, conscious of the fact that you felt hurt or that you were afraid of being hurt or perhaps afraid of hurting someone else.

This new awareness is of great importance in helping you to become truly conscious of what you no longer want for yourself and therefore what you want in its place. However, remember that the goal of this exercise is not to make you take blame or feel guilty or hit yourself over the head because you were in reaction mode that particular day. In fact this can only benefit you if you are able to feel gratitude for becoming more aware and if you give yourself the right to still be unable, FOR THE TIME BEING, to be what you want to be.

Let's suppose that one day you realize you have barely eaten all day, that you haven't even thought about eating. Later on, toward the end of the day, you start eating cookies and find you can't stop, and you don't even know how many you are eating. After checking the control behaviours that signify the various wounds, you notice that this behaviour is related to the wounds of rejection and injustice. You start to reflect about it and realize that you rejected yourself for a good part of the day. Perhaps you were afraid of being late with a certain task you had to complete and then being criticized by your superior? Or you were hard on yourself because you didn't feel up to the demands of a certain situation? Or maybe you started the same project over and over, without ever being satisfied with your work, because it was never good enough in your own estimation?

What is important here is to take the time to ask yourself at what moment you rejected yourself or were afraid of being rejected by another person or hated yourself for rejecting someone. Everything we experience in life, whether pleasant or unpleasant, is reproduced as a triangle.

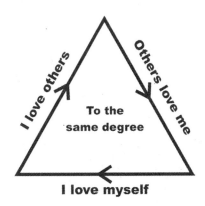

When two wounds are involved, as with the example given above, you will see that by working with one wound, the connections will easily be made with the other.

You can now establish the link between your way of eating on that particular day and what you experienced. Since you were rejecting yourself, you did not consider yourself important enough to be nourished and you didn't even think of eating. Toward the end of the day, you lost control, because your wound of injustice had been touched. Translation: you are very unjust toward yourself. Either you are controlling yourself – not enough food – or you are losing control – too much food. This is a good indicator of injustice toward yourself.

Remember that psychological research has shown that in general we are aware of barely 10% of what is going on inside us. We allow our ego to prevent us from being more conscious. Your first reaction may be one of denial. You might point out, *But no, I didn't experience any rejection today...* or *I did not accuse myself of anything.* This type of denial is one of the strategies the ego uses to keep us from becoming aware of our wounds. That way, it can continue to manage our life, convincing itself that it knows our needs better than we do, and is able to prevail over and over.

If you sometimes find it difficult to make the connection between the wound and the things that have happened to you that day or the day before, don't force the issue; However, don't close the door of your conscience either. You can ask your inner God to help you discover in what situation your wound was activated. After that, forget this request and busy yourself with another activity. The answer, very often, comes to us spontaneously, when we are not looking for it. Especially don't go searching too far back in time for the emotional trigger, because the reaction you express in the way you eat generally shows up within 24 hours of the event.

So, once you have been able to discover the rejection you experienced that day, reassure the suffering child inside you. Tell it that you are present with it and that it's quite human and normal to still have wounds that have not entirely healed. You can go on to reassure this little child by letting it know that you intend to heal these wounds one day, but that it is still going to take you a little while.

Finally you say THANK YOU to your inner God for having given you this realization today, through your observations about the way you eat. There must NEVER under any circumstances, be judgments, accusations, or criticisms on your part. I know it is easier said than done. Especially when you notice that your undesired behaviours have already been going on for quite some time, or when you thought you had really resolved certain things.

What you must also do is thank your body for being willing to co-operate with you by digesting, absorbing and eliminating everything you didn't need that day. Your body too has the need to be reassured. Explain to your body the journey you are on, that you are getting to know yourself through your dietary habits and that gradually you will be better able to listen to its needs. When your body feels that you truly accept yourself, that you **allow yourself to not yet be what you want to be**, it will be much more willing to co-operate with you.

It is like this with everything. **From the moment we accept ourselves in a certain state of being, a movement toward change is set in motion.** The less we accept ourselves, the less we change. The more we accept ourselves, the more things change. The ego cannot understand this statement because it only possesses mental comprehension that is limited to and tied to the past, while this statement is a spiritual reality, related to the present moment only. The ego is convinced that if you accept yourself while you are eating too much or not enough or food you do not need, this situation will persist and nothing will change. It believes that if you claim the right to be or to act a certain way, things will get worse and you will be even more unhappy. That's why your ego makes you feel guilty, hoping that you will continue to listen to it. It is convinced it is protecting you. The ego cannot understand that it is ONLY through acceptance that change can be initiated, not through control.

Healing your wounds

The explanation presented above describes a process you may engage in every evening after completing your daily journal when you observe that your way of eating did not correspond to your needs. If you wish to take the process further, and use your dietary habits as a means to heal your wounds, here are some additional stages to move into. However, you should know that it will require a little more time and, especially, the courage to let go, in order to face what is really going on inside you. It involves truly taking responsibility for yourself.

The biggest benefit to doing inner work is that by settling this matter of rejection and injustice definitively, future situations of this sort will no longer activate these two wounds. You will experience the situation in a totally different way and in a more objective, less emotionally charged, manner.

Emotions and accusations

The first stage consists of becoming aware of your experience.

Let us go back to the example mentioned above, the one where you have hardly eaten all day and later lost control, and then found that it was your wounds of rejection and injustice that were involved. What do you experience? What did you accuse yourself of in relation to the situations that took place that day? Did you hate yourself for being insufficiently prepared and waiting till the last minute to do this assignment? So, you accused yourself of being...

If this type of analysis is relatively new for you, it's a good idea to note down as you go along all the answers that come to you. You should note accusations to do with your BEING only. For example, I judged myself as BEING incompetent, too slow, a failure, a coward (because I did not dare to put in requests to my boss), abrasive with my colleagues at work...

How did you feel when the situation was occurring and how do you feel when you are reviewing the day? Find as many emotions and feelings as possible when writing: *I feel let down... frustrated... disappointed ... worried...* And don't forget *anger* and *sadness.* We can always find them behind all the other emotions we experience.

In addition, when you carefully review your day, do you find you have accused other people? Is it possible you have reproached your boss for being too demanding, that you believe she could have given you more time or provided you with more assistance for your work – thus awakening your wound of injustice? Do not forget to note down accusations relating to BEING, when it comes to other persons also. For example, *I accused him or her of BEING unfair, demanding, insensitive to my problems, cold...*

This analysis can help you get in touch with the anger and guilt you felt during the day, after taking multiple accusations. Allow yourself to really feel each of your emotions. A good way is to observe in what location in your body you feel each of these emotions. Afterwards, give them the room they need for the time being. Instead of resisting these emotions or denying them, tell yourself that it is impossible to accuse or judge anyone or to accuse oneself, without experiencing anger and guilt. That's part of being human. It is only when we are able to observe a situation without perceiving it as good or bad – that is, without judgment of any kind – that we can spare ourselves all these emotions.

It is very likely that after that, you will notice that you accuse yourself of the same thing regarding your dietary habits as you do regarding different situations that arise during the day. You hate yourself, for instance, for not listening to your needs, for forgetting about yourself, for waiting too long before taking nourishment, etc. Moreover, we feel guilty about the way we eat to the same degree that we feel guilty about whatever made us eat that way.

Guilt

The subject of guilt has recurred frequently since the beginning of this book. That's because even though it may seem obvious that guilt is the main reason why so many people have trouble letting go and listening to their needs, it remains nevertheless true that a great many people are not aware of the extent of their own guilt feelings.

Despite the fact that I talk about guilt and responsibility in all my workshops, lectures and books, I still feel the need to remind people of this notion. It is not only very important: it is essential for any permanent transformation, on all levels, but particularly in matters of the heart or in the spiritual sphere.

How often have I heard the numerous excuses people give, unaware that, as they do so, they are denying their feeling of guilt! I do not feel guilty, I'm just being careful not to gain weight... I am big like the other women in my family so I have no choice... I just don't want to make my wife unhappy as she goes to so much trouble to cook tasty meals for me, I just please myself, that's all, and I don't feel guilty about it... If they feel the need to defend themselves that way, guilt is the reason.

Once, on a cruise, my husband and I were assigned to the same dinner table of eight every evening. There was in our group a very slim, I would even say skinny, woman, who was accompanied by her VERY obese husband. She kept on making rude remarks about the heavy people who were walking around near our table. Her companion, for his part, did not seem to hear anything she said. It was easy to see that she did not accept heavy people, including herself should she inadvertently gain some weight. She perceived them as lax and weak-willed and believed they wouldn't be that heavy if they really desired not to be.

She stated that SHE never ate dessert, but I noticed that she picked at the food on her husband's plate quite a lot and that she drank a lot of wine – which contains sugar. I am sure she didn't even realize how often she ate from her husband's plate. One evening she told us that she had decided to give up bread and to reduce the amount of wine she consumed, for at least a month. I asked her if she felt guilty about eating or drinking them, or if she was abstaining from them for health reasons.

You should have seen her reaction! It was obvious she was shocked by my question. She stated tersely that given her age, it had been a very long time since she had felt any guilt. I checked with the other members of the group whether they sometimes felt guilty because I often heard them repeat that they had cheated during the day, that they would have to abstain in future, that they didn't have enough willpower, etc. Not one of them admitted that they experienced any guilt. It was as if this subject had suddenly become taboo, that it didn't concern them. I hastily changed the subject when I realized that these people refused to feel what was going on inside them. However, I could not help but listen and observe for the rest of the cruise and you cannot imagine the number of times when their actions and words demonstrated guilt. It was then that I really started to notice the prevalence of this issue around me, not only in North America but in many countries. It made me decide I would speak about guilt more often.

So, if this applies to you, do not be discouraged if you become aware, due to your alertness to what you are consuming, that there is more substance to your guilt feelings than you want to believe. If you are asking yourself why there is so much guilt in this world, here are two main reasons I have observed:

◆　We think that if we feel guilty, we won't do it again. We think this is true for others too and that's why we tend to make *them* feel guilty.

◆　We consider ourselves a good person because we think that if we do not experience guilt, we are bad or indifferent. We also think the same thing about others.

Now, do you understand why so many people constantly claim that they want to stop doing or eating this or that? For instance, *I am going to go on a diet starting next Monday so that I can "cheat" all weekend.* They make themselves believe and try to make others believe that they are not indifferent to their weight or their excess eating by having decided not to start again. When you feel guilty, making a decision, even a sincere one, will unfortunately not suffice.

Have you ever spoken those words at some point in your life? If you have, did you get the results you hoped for? Not really, right? Granted, you may have been able to control yourself for a period of time, but only to lose control again in this same area or another one. No one in the world can manage to control themselves indefinitely. We all have limits in that regard. On the other hand, the longer a person applies control, the greater the loss of control will be and sometimes all the more regrettable.

In the first two chapters of this book, you read about all the ways we use to control ourselves. By becoming conscious of what's going on in our life, through the use of the food journal that you are going to be filling in, you will see that most of the cases mentioned in those first two chapters generated guilt. As soon as we go against criteria that we learned, against what we were taught was good, what we were supposed to do, what was acceptable, nice, polite, considerate, loving…, guilt automatically settles in.

Take the example of the woman on the cruise. She was unconscious of what she was experiencing. She insisted to me that she believed a person was not guilty unless they had done something reprehensible, really bad, like theft or murder, etc. What she does not know is that our experience of mild or moderate guilt on a day-to-day basis turns out to be much more harmful than great guilt experienced occasionally during a lifetime. Why is that? Because in the case of major guilt, when someone is found guilty, it is much easier for that person to become aware of it, to face it, to finally deal with it, which is not the case in the example of that woman.

However, do not be surprised or alarmed if, as you become more aware, you regularly feel guilt. Instead of hating yourself for that, it is more important to be happy that you feel it. For, as long as we refuse to discover and feel what we are living, the same situation just repeats endlessly. As soon as you become aware of feeling guilty, the next stage is to check what are the fears that assail you in that situation. That's the stage that allows you to feel your suffering, allows you to develop more compassion toward yourself.

Fears for yourself

What did I fear for myself today in this situation? What am I afraid of as I review my day? Those are examples of questions to ask yourself. Let's go back to the example of rejection and injustice used earlier. The answer to those questions could be, *I was afraid I wasn't up to the job ... afraid of being fired ... afraid of making people laugh at me ... of being ridiculed ... at this moment I am afraid I will never learn to have more self-esteem ... I'm afraid others will notice how great my lack of self-confidence is, that I am weak and not very resourceful ... that they will discover I am not what they thought ...*

The important thing here is to bring out and note down all the fears that arise in you. If this type of exercise is new for you, it is possible that at first very few fears will present themselves. You might even think that you don't have any. If this happens, I suggest you give yourself the necessary time to put all these new theories into practice. Gradually, it will be less painful for you to face what you are actually experiencing. Everything gets easier and faster with practice, right? You will see how much easier it gets when you can give yourself permission to be human in the presence of fears. **Everyone has fears, without exception.** Our *raison d'être* on this earth is not to get rid of all our fears or to ignore them, but to be able to allow ourselves to have them, without judging or criticizing ourselves for being weak... dependent... vulnerable...

Now that you have gone through the stages involved in becoming conscious of the wounds activated on a particular day, by paying attention to your dietary habits and what you subsequently experienced (emotions, accusations, fears, etc.), there is just the final stage that remains: accepting yourself and loving yourself as you are IN THE MOMENT.

In order to do this, you must begin by taking responsibility for yourself. It is the only way I know of to break the vicious circle of guilt.

Responsibility

What is real responsibility? This notion has two aspects that cannot be dissociated:

► Knowing that we are always in the process of creating our life by the choices and decisions we make, which include our reactions.

► Knowing that others create their life according to the choices and decisions *they* make, which include their reactions.

The ultimate test that lets you determine whether you are truly responsible is to observe your ability to assume all the consequences of your decisions, actions and reactions, without blaming others, as well as your ability to let others assume the consequences of their choices and reactions without blaming yourself.

So, that is how you can transform guilt into responsibility, thanks to your food habits. Returning to the earlier example, when you become aware that you feel guilty for neglecting to take nourishment in the first place and later, for eating too many cookies, or basically, for going from one extreme to the other, you probably tell yourself, like most people, that you absolutely must turn over a new leaf.

But you know full well that you have repeated the same thing to yourself a thousand times.

Becoming responsible means noting your actions and reactions and reminding yourself that you have the right to act or do as you wish in life, while recognizing that there are always consequences to assume. So, I invite you to take a few moments to note what the positive and negative consequences are of depriving yourself and then going overboard.

Yes, I did say positive. It is possible that you considered it more important to finish your duties than it was to eat. It may also be that the cookies helped you to relax at the time, that they provided you with a comfort that you did not know how to find in any other way at that particular moment, as you were demanding too much of yourself. After noting all the consequences, it is purely up to you to decide if this behaviour brings you more happiness and satisfaction than worries and problems. And it is for you to recognize that only you can assume the consequences and that there is no one else in your life who can tell you what to do, what to eat, what to drink.

I fear you may have the same reaction as many other people, that when you read these lines, you right away say to yourself, But I cannot allow myself to behave that way and especially not to eat all those cookies; then I would risk keeping this bad habit, especially always eating more cookies, which are my weakness… This is a totally normal and human reaction. The ego cannot understand the notion of acceptance and responsibility. All it knows comes from what it has learned: if you give yourself the right, you will always continue the same process, risking making the situation worse if you don't decide to get rid of this bad habit.

So then you have to talk to that part of you – your ego – that believes in this false notion. Explain to it that until now, by following what it believes, nothing has changed anyway and that as far as you are concerned, it's time to try something new. You must above all reassure your ego that it will not have to assume the consequences of your decision. You alone will be doing that. Your ego, by way of the little voices that you constantly hear in your head, wants to help you because it is convinced that it is acting in your best interests.

Thanks to your diet, you have in your possession a formidable tool for learning how to dialogue with your ego, which is an excellent way to become once again the sole master of your life. When you take a decision and you accept ahead of time that you are assuming all the consequences relating to it, **even if this decision does not meet one of your deeper needs**, do you realize that YOU ARE THE MASTER DIRECTING YOUR LIFE at that particular moment? Why? I want to stress one more time that you are not obliged to explain yourself to anyone. Besides, it is by living all kinds of experiences and by accepting them that we sharpen our discernment and become more conscious of our true needs.

Let us suppose that you decide to continue to behave in the same way and to eat lots of cookies, but this time while being more alert to the consequences. When the consequences become too hard to take, be assured that you will find it easy to decide to eat fewer of them until you reach a point where you don't need them at all anymore. While you are eating them, you know that you would like one day to be able to show kindness to yourself in another way, but that for now, you are not able to behave differently.

You will only be able to see the validity of this theory when you have really experienced it. **True knowing can only come from experience, not from mere information.**

Staying with our example above, here is an excellent way of finding out whether you still feel guilty or if you are really taking responsibility for yourself. Observe whether you are able to go overboard with the cookies – or something else – in the presence of others, without feeling obliged to offer an excuse. Check whether others are able to watch you having all those cookies, without making you feel guilty. If not, if you feel some kind of uneasiness, it is a sign that you still feel guilty. But, whatever you do, do not despair at this. Taking responsibility for yourself involves a big learning curve. The great majority of people never learned in childhood or adolescence what taking responsibility really means and, if they did, probably did not learn how to apply it. You will have to remind yourself frequently that in reality no one is guilty of anything. We are all in the process of trying out many things in order to discover what is best for us, what is more intelligent for us.

Loving yourself means giving yourself the right to undertake this learning process, whether you succeed or not. Just think back to the day you wanted to learn to ride a bicycle. Didn't you find it normal to fall and to have to start over several times before you could balance yourself? Did you consider yourself a bad person or stupid because you didn't succeed on the first try? This applies to any new things we want to learn. However, when we are dealing with beliefs connected with our wounds, it will require more time, patience and perseverance to reach our goal, because we have been dragging these wounds around with us for many lifetimes. The main thing is to bring out our good intentions and especially to be able to note constant improvement over time.

When you observe that you are still feeling guilty, here's what you can do: instead of being down on yourself for this, take the time to check the degree of guilt you feel at present, compared to the guilt you felt before you started to make changes. For example, if currently you would rate the strength of your guilt feelings, on a scale of one to ten, as being a five, while before it was a nine, you can see that you have made progress. This brief exercise can be very helpful in preventing discouragement and also in keeping our expectations realistic. If, on the other hand, you find you feel even more guilt, it's just that you are more aware of it and it is only this awareness that can lead you to acceptance and thus to healing.

By becoming a responsible person in the area of food, you are already setting in motion the same process in the other areas of your life where you feel guilty. In the example mentioned above, you will gradually become aware that you are demanding too much of yourself at your work and that you are accusing yourself of things of which you are not in any way guilty. You will see also that your fears and accusations are not bringing you the beneficial results you aspire to in life. You will learn that even if you do not live up to the expectations of your superior, for example, you will know how to deal with that at the appropriate time and you will be able to assume the consequences.

Making peace with
your parents

In addition to accepting the behaviours influenced by your wounds, which you do by applying the responsibility principle, if you wish to advance further on this path of acceptance, your life can be transformed even more rapidly. However, this stage would require that you set aside more time to be alone with yourself for introspective work and, afterwards, arrange to meet with certain people in order to bring this spiritual work to fruition.

Let us summarize by returning to the same example. Up to this point, you have become conscious

  a)   that you have not listened to your body's needs in the way that you eat;
  b)   of the connection between your dietary habits and the wounds of rejection and injustice activated that day;
  c)   of the emotions and feelings experienced that day, especially guilt;
  d)   of the accusations made toward yourself and your superior;
  e)   of the fears that dwell in you;
  f)   that you must become a responsible person rather than nourishing a feeling of guilt.

The next stage consists of making the connection with your parents or those who had a strong influence on your education.

When you criticize another person, you can also make the connection with your parent of the same sex as that person. However, if the criticism is directed toward someone in the professional field – as in the above example –, you can make the connection with anyone of that sex who taught you during your childhood or adolescence.

When you criticize yourself, you should know that this attitude also relates to the parent of the same sex as you and involves the same attribute for which they criticized themselves. Ask yourself in what circumstances you criticized this parent for being… [whatever you discovered earlier]. In other words, you have to be aware that this parent criticized themselves in the same way. In fact, they experienced the same emotions as you – associated with the same wound – with the same degree of pain with their own parent as with you. This stage should help you open your heart and develop compassion toward this parent and toward yourself.

Referring to the triangle I explained earlier, it shows you that if you accuse another person, that person accuses you of the same thing and you behave in a similar fashion toward yourself. When it is yourself you are judging or accusing, you can likewise use this triangle. In that case, someone else is accusing you of the same thing and, for your part, you repeat this behaviour when they are like you.

Take a few moments then to feel the suffering that all of these emotions together associated with your wounds have made you experience, as explained earlier in this chapter.

Now that you are learning and recognizing that your parent experienced the same degree of suffering as you, is it easier to have compassion and to allow them to have acted as they did toward you, knowing they could not have done otherwise at that time given their own wounds? Give yourself all the time you need to reach this openness of heart.

Once this work of compassion has been done, all that remains is to share it with that parent. That is the stage where you will be able to discover the extent of your acceptance of that parent and of yourself. If this last step, called the stage of reconciliation and true forgiveness, is difficult for you, it's because the pain associated with this situation is intense. It is a sign that the journey of acceptance is not yet completed, that your ego still has a hold over you and wants to convince you that this parent or you yourself should take blame. By continuing to put yourself in the skin of this parent, you will see that little by little, your heart will open and you will finally be able to share with your parent what you have discovered.

In the area of food, it is also possible to make peace with your parents, by noting whether you judged them in any way with respect to how they ate, or the way they nourished your three bodies – physical, emotional and mental – when you were young.

There is nothing in the world that can help you more to direct yourself toward what you want to be than this process of self-acceptance and acceptance of others. It is especially recommended in relation to behaviours and states of being that you experience in the moment and that have become too harmful for you to tolerate any longer. You know now that nothing changes by your staying in control mode. Only true acceptance can obtain an effect that is as remarkable and lasting.

You will know that your wounds are on the way to being healed the moment you give yourself the right to sometimes reject, abandon, humiliate, betray and be unfair with others, especially those closest to you. Your wounds grow to the degree that you do not accept who you are in the moment, with your weaknesses, your limits and your disabilities and, equally importantly, with the positive aspects of who you are.

Being what you want to be

One method that is often suggested for becoming conscious of what you want is to ask yourself the following question: *The fact that I am...* (Repeat what you have judged yourself to be in this situation) *prevents me from being what?* The answer to this question tells you what you want for yourself in this type of situation. For example, *the fact that I am incompetent prevents me from being confident and taking initiative and having more self-esteem...* Thus your deep desire is to be confident and to take initiative in order to have greater self-esteem.

Take the time to re-live your day in thought, experiencing it the way that you would like to live it now, if it were to manifest itself again. Visualize that day by imagining the person you want to be one day. Let the images that arise in you come to the surface. This is a fantastic exercise for setting in motion what you want to see happen. On the other hand, don't be disappointed if what you desire does not manifest itself right away. It may indeed come about immediately, but it is just as likely that everything will happen gradually. Only the future can tell.

I know that after doing this type of introspective work on acceptance, if ever the same or a similar situation were to arise, you would not experience it in the same way, and especially, you would experience it with less emotional and mental pain. Moreover, you will be pleasantly surprised to notice yourself behaving more in tune with what you want to become. Staying in contact with what you want to BE is enough: if you remain alert, the thoughts, ideas and actions will present themselves on their own.

Repeat to yourself often what your desire is, what it is you want and what you want to be. Write it down everywhere. Repetition produces new connections in our brain. The big corporations discovered this fact a very long time ago and make large-scale use of it in their repeated advertisements. As long as you are constantly talking to yourself, which is a form of autosuggestion, you might as well repeat to yourself things that you like to hear and that will help you.

When you do not instantly become what you want to be or you are not behaving in accordance with what you want, remember to repeat this to yourself: *It would be preferable or desirable for me to be... and I will get there, but for now, this is not the case. I must give myself time.*

Accepting your weight

We have been focusing on acceptance since the beginning of this chapter, but if at the moment that you are reading these lines, you are among those who do not like themselves at all with their current weight – too thin, too fat –, the same exercises of awareness and acceptance are needed.

What wound is activated by this weight problem? Once the wound is identified, you proceed to the same stages mentioned in the section "Making peace with your parents", starting with the things of which you accuse yourself and/or others, then moving through the subsequent stages.

On the other hand, some people claim they couldn't have hated their parents, because neither of them had a weight problem. If this applies to you, don't stop at the bodily appearance. The answer lies in how you or they felt. That's what matters, what touches your being. So, the fact of being heavy, how does that make you feel? Observe all the emotions that well up. And then ask yourself *how am I judging myself* or *what am I accusing myself of*? Let's say you judge yourself as being weak or spineless, as being too compulsive, as being hypocritical or dishonest – because you hide when you eat. Check when you accused your parents of being like that. It might very well be in an area other than food.

What I am really saying is to focus your attention not on your physical appearance but on what is hidden beyond that appearance, that is to say, in the emotional and mental dimensions. I assure you that as you undertake inner transformation, it will impact on your physical body.

How do you know what you need to be more attentive to? Suppose you have learned that when you look at yourself, you consider yourself ugly, repulsive, heavy and slow. You ask yourself the question presented above, which I repeat here: *The fact of being...* (Here, repeat what you have just discovered) *prevents me from being, from having what?* If the answer is that it prevents you from being comfortable... flexible... confident... free... graceful... you are discovering what you really want to be. Draw up a list then of the behaviours you could adopt in your life that would help you to become that person. That way, instead of putting all the emphasis on your weight, you divert your attention toward what you would like to be from now on.

Place this list in a prominent place and, every day, take a step or do one thing that will help you be what you want to be. For instance, if you want to be comfortable, you could make sure to wear a comfortable item of clothing that day. Or it might be to make sure you have a well-padded chair if you need to be sitting in one place for several hours. In addition to your actions, you can be more comfortable in the words you speak, in your thoughts or your decisions, by being genuine. For example, when you are preparing to make a decision, you can take a few moments to ask yourself if your are comfortable with this decision, thus helping your soul to progress, to be happier and to orient itself toward what it wants to be.

I have noticed that often those who carry excess weight are people who have developed the bad habit of taking on an excess load – generally of an affective nature – from those close to them. They often take too much onto their shoulders. Indeed, they look after the needs of others while they neglect their own. If this sounds like you, you can ask those close to you (but are not dependent on you) if they would be kind enough to let you know when you behave that way. The people that you see as taking advantage of you often, or expecting too much of you, behave that way only because you let them. They quickly realized that you are willing to take on their problems and they take advantage of it. This is another way for you to become conscious of the reasons for your excess weight. You can also create a sign that you put in various places around your house to remind you to take responsibility for yourself and to let others take responsibility for themselves. So, there you have two actions that can definitely help you to take a new direction into the future.

Accepting others, whatever their weight

Accepting excess weight in someone you love seems as difficult as accepting it in yourself, sometimes even more so. Surprising, isn't it? This may prove to be the case in a situation where you have always controlled or paid attention to your weight and then find that you have a child or spouse who seems prone to obesity.

How many moms have not approached me about this, seeming completely helpless – dads feel this way too sometimes, although they show it less. These moms simply could not accept seeing their lovely daughter grow heavier-looking with each passing year. Most of them reacted in identical fashion, by adopting a directive type of behaviour to motivate their daughter to pay attention to her weight, in other words, to control herself.

What they didn't know was that this is the worst method a mother could adopt. Imagine a young girl of eleven or twelve, quite chubby, whose mom tells her things like: *You are so pretty, honey, but you know, if you keep gaining weight like this, none of the boys are going to be interested in you later on... I've bought you a little book to help you keep track of your calories... Stop that snacking, aren't you embarrassed? You just finished your dinner less than half an hour ago!... If I had eaten the way you do when I was gaining weight during my teens, can you imagine what I would look like today? Right. Big as a whale or like your*

179

grandma... You know, my dear, I know it's none of my business, but don't you think you should go on a diet? ...

All this young girl hears is that her mother doesn't love her as she is and it is only when she is slimmer that she will be able to feel loved or accepted by her. And when Mom congratulates her daughter on those occasions when she has been able to control herself, what the daughter will have learned and retained in her belief system is that in life one must control oneself in order to be loved. Her mom does not realize that she is influencing her daughter to further strengthen the masks associated with her wounds. We know that as soon as we control ourselves, we are not ourselves, but have donned the mask associated with the awakened wound. The masks do more harm than the excess weight.

If you experience this type of problem with one of your children or your partner or your parent, for instance, you must surely be asking yourself, *But what do you do with someone who doesn't have any will power? If nobody talks to them about it, their problem will get worse and one day it will be too late to do anything about it. I only want to help. I have no intention of hurting someone I love.*

It is true that all the moms who have approached me on this issue came only with good intentions. I have to remind you here that **the power of intention can only work for oneself**. So, even if you have the best intentions in the world, you cannot force another person. No one has this power. Besides, we should not try to avail ourselves of this power. It shows a lack of respect. A very good example to illustrate this concept is the donkey whose master was determined to make it drink. Try as he might, by pulling, pushing, forcing its mouth open to take water, there was nothing the master could do to make the donkey drink if the donkey didn't want to. The master's good intentions, so to speak, had no effect on the desired outcome. Don't we always say, *You can lead a horse to water, but you can't make it drink?*

Accepting the other person as they are means leaving them free to make their own decisions and to assume the related consequences. To go back to the example of the mother and her daughter, here's an approach that might be helpful. She could sit down with her daughter and share with her the fact that she has noticed her daughter is increasingly gaining weight, that this may reverse on its own later, or it may continue, but no one can tell what the future will bring.

Then, she could ask her daughter how she feels about the fact that she is heavier than many of her peers. Does it interfere with her relationships at school, her relationships with her friends? On a physical level, does it get in the way of her performance in sports? The important thing is to get her to talk about it and especially to talk about what she feels. Next, she might ask her daughter if she would be willing to draw up a list – on her own or with her mom – of all the possible consequences for her, if she were nevertheless to gain more weight.

Once you have taken stock, Mom checks in with her daughter to find out how she feels about assuming these consequences, explaining to her that no one else can do this for her. If you decide to take this approach with another person, the best way to know if you are acting from the heart at the moment when you want to help them is to observe their reaction.

If the young girl replies that she couldn't care less about the consequences, that she's not *that* heavy and that, after all, it's *her* body and it's no one else's business, it means that she felt that Mom had expectations and was determined to get results from her suggestions. The youth of today have a much stronger sense of their own psychological power than the previous generation. They refuse to let themselves be controlled by their parents or educators. They can sense very quickly whether their parents are trying to control them or just want to help them, coming from their heart, not set on getting specific results.

Why is this so? Because their need for respect is very strong. They have known since birth that as soon as someone tries to control or change another person, it shows a great lack of respect. All those who have been born with the energy of the age of Aquarius are much more conscious of this great need for respect. This energy began to be felt on Earth in the sixties and has been growing stronger and more powerful year by year ever since.

When young people are brought to look squarely at the consequences of their actions, they know intuitively that this notion of responsibility is fair and just.

We know we have truly integrated the true notion of responsibility when we are able to let others assume the consequences of their choices, decisions and reactions.

When a child feels that their parent is simply guiding them to become a responsible person and that, whatever decisions they make, their parent will be able to adjust, even if they do not agree, that child will listen much more to their parent's advice.

Therefore, you'll be able to tell right away, just from the other person's reaction, that you do not feel responsible for their decisions. But if you decide to take responsibility for them and you give advice to avoid feeling guilty, the result will be that the other person feels blame has been cast on them by your advice. Indeed, they will feel right away that you have expectations. You want them to listen to you, to change, so that you will not feel guilty. You act this way more out of fear for yourself than out of a desire to help the other person meet their needs.

As soon as you have expectations following some advice given to someone, it indicates a condition, a "non-acceptance" on your part. How do you feel when someone suggests something to you and you can feel right away that they have expectations? Even if they add that you can follow it or not, you know, don't you, that that person will be disappointed if you don't take their advice into account. If you are like most people, you must surely have no desire whatsoever to listen to such advice.

It is sad to have to admit how many of us have expectations, that is to say, we wish to control the result for the other person. For, very often, the advice we give others is quite valid initially, but rarely gets listened to in the end. Generally speaking, if the advice given was not asked for, it's the one giving it who probably has the greater need to follow it. This must be because if we can't control ourselves and make ourselves perfect, then we want to try and make someone else perfect!

In the situation where you want to help someone suffering from excess weight, if you doubt that you have let go and are capable of feeling fine with whatever decision the other person will make, it's a good idea to ask them if they think you have really let go and if they feel completely free to make whatever decision they want. How can you know the needs of that person's soul and what they need to learn in this life? Maybe they need to live this life as an obese person in order to work on their wounds? This is why no one in the world has the right to decide for another.

As the mother of a child who tends to gain weight, you can do your part by buying healthy foods that are more nutritious and provide a lot of energy. Your child won't need to eat as much. It was while my children were still teenagers, and I was starting my research about food and the link between the physical and psychic bodies, that I came to realize I was buying many foods and drinks that didn't provide any energy at all. Quite the opposite! A huge quantity of energy was being required to digest, absorb and eliminate all these foods that were useless to the body. For example, when my kids were thirsty, they always drank sweetened juices. So, I bought an appliance that improved the quality of our water. The reason they had not been drinking tap water is that it simply wasn't drinkable as it tasted so much of chemicals. I understood perfectly when they said, *Finally, water that tastes good!*

Looking at your ability to respect the needs of others is an important factor in becoming aware of your ability to respect your own needs.

Listening to the needs of your three "bodies"

The three bodies – physical, emotional and mental – each have very specific needs. If you do not nourish them adequately, it will be impossible for you to feel good about yourself. I am using the opportunity of this book to review them with you, so it will be easier for you to keep your life goals clearly in mind and be able one day to realize them, giving yourself along the way the time you need to get there.

Starting with the **physical body**, the five essential elements it needs have already been mentioned at the beginning of the book. Trusting your body fully, acknowledging that it knows exactly what it needs, will remove a huge burden from you each day. You will notice that after several weeks of practice asking yourself the question, *What do I feel like eating?*, you are able to listen to your needs more easily and more quickly. My fondest wish for you is that you fall more and more in love with the intelligence of your body, which knows exactly what it needs at every instant. You will recall that in addition to food, water, breathing and physical activity (these last two were discussed in the previous chapter), the physical body needs rest, which of course includes sleep. Actually, this need is equally essential for the emotional and mental bodies.

The biggest excuse people give for not getting enough rest is usually time. This is really foolish and does not make sense because, after resting, you accomplish twice as much work in the same amount of time and you are able to do it more efficiently. All you have to do is try it out for yourself to check out the truth of what I have just said. Here is a wise decision you could adopt as of today: take rest, in addition to taking some kind of recreation that really appeals to you. Time is not something we possess but an energy that is available to everyone. We can adapt our use of time according to our priorities at any given moment. **If you do not devote time to looking after your health in the present, you will have to take time to look after your illnesses later.** What do you choose? For example, just 15 or 30 minutes of relaxation is very often enough to give us that extra burst of energy we need.

With respect to sleep, your body's needs will vary, depending on the activities you engage in during the day. After trying different methods, here is the one I discovered that has been working very well for me for many years. In the evening, I mentally review what I have planned for the next day and I ask my body to let me know at what time I should go to bed. As soon as I feel my eyelids grow heavy, that's the signal. However, don't forget that if you do not listen to the signal your body gives you, it will gradually stop sending you that information and you will soon lose the ability to understand its message, just like in the example about listening to your body when it is telling you it's time to stop eating.

Now, with respect to the **emotional body**, it was created to feel, to resonate, to be aroused and to desire a life of happiness, joy, beauty and inner peace. In short, it wants to feel well and happy, not stressed and frightened, not be feeling sorry for itself over its fate. Let me clarify. Here are several causes of stress: being too perfectionist – believing we are responsible for the happiness of others (therefore, feeling guilty if they are not happy) – dramatizing events – wanting to control everything – believing that in order to be

186

successful, we must work hard and not take time out to enjoy ourselves or relax on a regular basis – identifying ourselves with what we do or have (for example, I'm a failure, because I went bankrupt) – wanting to live up to the expectations of others – demanding a lot of ourselves – fear of being egotistical – controlling ourselves constantly in order not to gain weight…

Your emotional body, asks you instead to count your blessings every day, to thank yourself as well as others and to have gratitude toward Life for everything this day has given you. It asks you to compliment rather than criticize yourself.

It also needs to have goals, to have things to look forward to, on a daily basis. When you are keen to get up in the morning and you picture something interesting, it is an indication that your emotional body is happy. The body produces energy constantly and this energy needs to be used by an activity you are enthusiastic about. The best example is that of a child who is bored, complaining, and in a bad mood. Find something interesting for them to do, something they like, and you will see them light up instantly.

As for your **mental body**, it needs to be nourished with additional knowledge to stimulate the brain, to live new experiences in order to learn and to stay alert. This is the body that helps you think, analyze, and organize and also maintain your memory. It needs to entertain beneficial thoughts and to live in the present.

If, on the contrary, you don't want to learn anything new, you will become a person of habit and your beliefs will direct your life. You will live mainly in the past, which ends up paralyzing you, rather than helping you to improve your present.

Find your own way to acquire new knowledge that will feed your mental body, whether through reading, workshops, television, or the Internet... or by simply taking the time to listen carefully to the people around you. At the end of the day, just saying thank you for whatever new thing you have learned that day will help you to be conscious that you have nourished your mental body. However, the new knowledge you acquire should help you to be what you want to be or to become. If it is not used, it will quickly be forgotten.

Meditation

Another excellent method for connecting you with yourself and discovering your needs is meditation. This is an excellent habit and you should waste no time getting started on it. All the great spiritual traditions have been talking about it from earliest times.

For about twenty years now, more and more research has been producing interesting scientific conclusions about meditation. In fact, they have been able to show that brain patterns change considerably in people who have been meditating regularly for some years. From the lines on the graphs, they have observed that the different regions of the brain oscillate in harmony and are synchronized when these people are in their meditative state. The more people engage in frequent meditation, the more there appears to be a cumulative effect of this harmony and the effects of meditation become increasingly prolonged between meditation periods.

Certain researchers have even established that the regions of the brain associated with joy and a positive outlook were more active. We have also known for a long time that people who meditate regularly have a much more active immune system than those who do not.

For my part, I started to meditate about thirty years ago and I have noted several benefits from it. To be specific, it has helped me develop my concentration, be able to work efficiently even when there is noise around me, for example, from teenagers in the house. The greatest benefit I have been able to notice is reduced fear and anxiety. I used to have a great deal of anxiety, especially during the first years of my Listen To Your Body School. I have also noticed that in the hours following my meditation, wonderful spontaneous inspirations as well as answers to my questions often come to me.

People often ask, How should I know what type of meditation to do? There are so many ways of meditating that are suggested out there! My answer to them is, Why don't you try out at least a few of them and find out which one works best for you? Furthermore, there is information on this subject available on the Internet, in books and through workshops. I tried several kinds of meditation in the first few years and my preference is for the kind that uses observation, which I will share with you here.

WHEN should you meditate? Ideally, at sunrise. If that is not convenient for you, meditate at the time that works best for you. But remember that the more the day advances, the more your thoughts will start bubbling up in you, making it harder to remain in observation mode. Moreover, it is suggested that you not meditate after your evening meal, but do something relaxing instead.

HOW? You sit down in a chair, with your back as straight as possible and your feet flat on the floor. (This position is not intended to be a relaxing one where you can stretch out.) Then you close your eyes and place your hands on your knees. After three deep breaths, you breathe normally – as indicated earlier in this book – and you keep your attention focused on your breathing, all the while trying to observe that the air that enters you brings you peace, calm and health and that your exhalations help to free you of the stress and toxins that have built up inside you.

WHERE? It is recommended that you create a personal meditation corner, a space where it will be possible to have peace and quiet. You could put out a picture that you find inspiring, light a candle to create a calming atmosphere. You could also play peaceful music as additional support to help quieten your mind.

FOR HOW LONG? If you are not accustomed to meditation, you can begin with fifteen or twenty minutes a day, increasing to thirty minutes or an hour if you feel comfortable doing so. Consider this time as being precious, time just for you; it is an opportunity to be alone in communion with yourself.

The comment I get the most frequently is, *I have often sat down to meditate but I do not manage, however, to stop thinking.* Don't worry, this is completely normal. There are very few people who can go more than ten minutes without thinking. So, do not expect to reach that stage in the first few days. You can even begin with five minutes a day, increasing the duration gradually over the weeks. Indeed, we all have a long way to go before we achieve the mastery of meditation of the great Tibetan monks.

To meditate is to observe your thoughts and feelings. As soon as a thought arises in your consciousness, like, *I must not forget to call the dentist today to cancel my appointment*, you observe it, pronouncing the word THOUGHT and you let it pass knowing you can come back to it after your meditation. You do this for any thought or any feeling that comes along. If you suddenly feel sadness, while thinking about a person with whom you had an argument, you observe this and pronounce FEELING and let it pass. It could be FEAR, GUILT, ANGER... You only say one word to designate what has just arisen and then allow it to pass. In the same way, you note any physical SENSATION that occurs in your body, like ITCH or PAIN or HEAT, etc. With practice and perseverance, I can promise you that meditation will become easier and more pleasant.

To differentiate clearly between "thinking" and "observing", I like using the following example. Imagine that you are sitting by the riverside and you see a lot of debris floating on the water – pieces of wood, garbage... If you simply observe, you note what you see and you watch it pass. There is no mental activity at all. But if you think, you start to analyze and ask yourself questions like, *Where might all that garbage be coming from? What kind of thoughtless people are polluting this beautiful river?*

Afterwards, you can always reflect on certain aspects of what has come to you during the meditation. But while you are meditating, you must observe as much as possible. It is this phenomenon – the state of observation – that produces such beneficial consequences, often even more so than sleep.

Respecting yourself and loving yourself

As you can see, all the methods indicated in this book are intended to help you know yourself better and love yourself more. The more you put them into practice, the easier it will be for you to listen to the needs of your body. Feeling loved and respected, your body will give back to you one hundredfold and team up with you. If there are occasions when you have to ask your body to make available to you a surplus of energy or endurance, it will be glad to co-operate with you, knowing how much help you will give it in return. As well, you are going to realize how much your diet will change and be transformed; because you will love yourself so much that it will start to pain you to be careless about the way you nourish your body.

I know that most of us are too demanding and even intransigent with ourselves, and by that very fact, that we have a hard time accepting ourselves. It seems we never live up to our own standards. We never think that doing our best is enough, far from it. As perfectionists, we either exhaust ourselves trying to do it all perfectly and achieve our goals, or we become paralyzed. We might even go so far as to give up entirely for fear of failure. *If I do nothing, I can be sure I won't make a mistake,* we tell ourselves. If you recognize yourself as this type of person, the following sentence can help you to accept your limits. *I always do my best and I accept that it is impossible to do everything perfectly..*

A major cause of stress is the belief that we are respon-sible for the happiness of others. It is totally human to be sad when misfortune strikes a person we love. But it is not, however, beneficial to get stressed out, to engage in self-destructive behaviour when faced with a situation we can-not change, especially when it is someone else's situation. One day, I read the following sentence, which helps us to realize that each of us is responsible for our own decisions: *It's not that misfortune always besets the same poor people, it's just that there are people who find what they are look-ing for.* Indeed, there are people who, despite all the assis-tance you were able to lend them and all the emotions you went through on their behalf, continue constantly to attract misfortune.

These poor people believe – unknowingly – that it is the only way to get attention. And you, all that time? You think you are giving them love, when in reality, this is not so. When you insist on reforming another person's life, it is generally to be loved in return and acknowledged. This shows then that you do not love yourself and do not recog-nize the special person that you are. You need to be loved by others in order to love yourself.

It will be a much smarter and more useful idea in future to give yourself all the love you need, because when you come down to it, no one else can do that for you. Loving yourself is very simple. All you have to do is give yourself the right to be what you are at every instant, without judg-ment or criticism on your part. When you are capable of loving in this manner, I can assure you that the help you will decide to offer others after that will be very different and more appreciated. You will help them by respecting their needs while at the same time respecting yourself. You will not insist. You will be able to discern whether this person really wants to obtain help. This form of help will be given out of love and not out of fear of not being loved and will prove to be so much more energizing for you, instead of exhausting and harmful.

With respect to diet, **loving yourself** means giving yourself the right to not be perfect, to not always listen to your dietary needs. It is to accept being human with limitations and needs. **Respecting yourself** means taking the time to ask yourself whether the choice you are making answers one of your needs. In this way, even if you authorize yourself to not always do things that are liable to meet a need, that doesn't mean that this same behaviour will continue for the rest of your life. It is only TODAY that you are allowing yourself not to listen to your needs, while at the same time reminding yourself that you also want to learn to have greater respect for your body. Let's take the example of a family gathering. Perhaps you overdo it with food and drinks. At a certain point, you become aware that you did not listen to your needs during this party. But by telling yourself that it was for TODAY, this attitude will not persist, and it will be easier to allow yourself this behaviour. You know, furthermore, that you are the only one who assumes the consequences of all your actions.

Respecting yourself also means knowing when to say NO to certain foods and certain persons. It means remembering that your body has been created perfectly for your fulfillment in this life. By listening to its needs, regardless of its size, colour or shape, it will always be there to help you. You need only do your best to meet its needs. Treat your body with all the dignity and love it deserves. The way you nourish it is but the reflection of the way you nourish the needs of your soul. Your eating habits help you become conscious of the degree of love and respect you have for yourself.

Having gone through that experience, I guarantee you an imminent transformation, which others will see in you very soon, when you have greater self-respect. In fact your family and friends will feel that you are someone to be respected, even if they are not conscious of the change.

Transformation and physical healing

I can further assure you that you will observe several physical transformations as you progress in adopting new behaviours with a view to listening to your needs. Your physical body will change in several ways. It is very possible that your body will be healed form numerous ailments and illnesses.

In all the years that I have been teaching at the Listen To Your Body School (since 1982), I have received thousands of testimonies to this effect, either sent to me by mail or told to me in person. Your physical body is only the reflection of what is happening on the emotional and mental levels. Consequently, your three bodies are transformed at the same time. They cannot be dissociated.

I am not claiming that you should not take care of your physical body when it is ill. You must look after it with the treatment of your choice. But if you decide to look after your other two bodies by modifying your way of thinking and living, then, thanks to your changed behaviour, you will have the pleasant surprise of seeing your physical body heals much faster.

The proactive approach that you are taking now, by loving yourself enough to listen to your needs, has been shown to be the most effective way to avoid numerous physical problems later on. For example, we often attract accidents when we are feeling guilty. It is a method we use subconsciously to punish ourselves when we find ourselves guilty. Remember that every time you control yourself, in any area at all, it is sign of guilt feelings. As you begin to control yourself less, you will notice that those guilt feelings also start diminishing – at the same rate. Don't you think you are a special enough person to deserve to live a happier and more harmonious life? It is totally up to you!

I urge you, therefore, to develop the habit of noting down in your daily journal the progress you make and everything you are proud of that day. This offers you a wonderful opportunity to manifest your love for yourself. Is that not a more agreeable and soul-nurturing way to end your day than feeling guilty and focusing on what you don't like about yourself? Afterwards, don't forget to reward yourself in areas other than food. Then, you will seek less and less to use food as a reward. It is always preferable to start the reward process with words. For example, you might congratulate yourself out loud for what you are and for what you have done today. Follow this up with a totally different type of reward and you will feel prompted to start or carry on with a new habit that is better for you!

Thank you, my body, for what you have helped me discover today. I come to know myself a little better each day and accept myself as I am.

196

Conclusion

Aide-mémoire & Conclusion

This *aide-mémoire* has been added for readers who are interested in keeping a daily food journal, as suggested in this book. Keeping a journal will help you achieve better and deeper self-knowledge far more rapidly.

This chapter has four clear objectives:

► To provide you with a model of the food journal to be kept daily. (However, it might be better and more practical for you to look up this model on the Web site www.lisebourbeau.com and to print up several copies.)

► To provide you, in addition, with a sample, mini-poster, that says AM I REALLY HUNGRY? This little visual reminder can be placed on your fridge or cupboard right at the start to get you into the habit of asking yourself this question. (This sheet can also be found on the above Web site).

► To remind you how to fill out the journal at the end of each day.

► To help you get to know yourself by checking the way you interpret what you note in your journal.

Remember that the SOLE PURPOSE of the daily exercise of completing this journal is to get to know yourself. If during the day you think: *I must not eat this second piece of cake because I am going to be ashamed to write that down in my journal tonight,* it would be preferable that you not fill out this journal because this behaviour represents an attitude of control. Thinking along the same lines, if when you are filling in the journal, you are inclined to lie about what you ate or drank, in case someone were to find your sheet, you do not have the right kind of motivation and this is another form of control.

Remember the title of this book: **Listen and Eat: STOP CONTROLLING YOURSELF**. Its intent is not to provoke more control. You must be motivated ONLY by the desire to know yourself, to be happy and to discover aspects of yourself that you did not know before and would not have become aware of if you had not completed this journal. You will find a sample copy of the journal at the end of this chapter.

How to complete the journal

Start with the first two columns. Note the time and what you ate and/or drank, beginning with the evening and ending with when you got up.

Next, you note down the number of glasses of water you drank that day.

For each time you ate or drank something, you note in the next column whether you were hungry (or thirsty) or not.

If you were hungry and you asked yourself if you felt like eating and if then you listened to your need, you put a checkmark in the column **Eat as needed**.

If you were hungry and you did not listen to your need, you put a checkmark in the appropriate following column(s).

If you were not hungry, check the column(s) that influenced you to eat or drink without needing to.

In the **Link** column, you note down everything you can remember about what happened that day and that could have influenced you to eat that particular way.

If you notice that you often forget to ask yourself the question *AM I REALLY HUNGRY?* before consuming something, I suggest you put up the mini-poster displaying this question in various places throughout the kitchen. You will then find it easier to complete your journal. You will know more quickly whether or not you were hungry for each food eaten and noted down.

To help you further, here is a review of how to interpret the various motivations for eating.

You are motivated by *PRINCIPLE* when you eat or drink influenced by the notion of good and evil or by fear. The following situations would come under this category:

♦ Fear of waste. Eating or drinking something (liquid or solid) before it goes bad, or before the Best Before date. Finishing your plate rather than throwing out what is too much for you. Even finishing other people's plates. Eating everything offered in the special deal, for example, the bread, soup, entrée and dessert, just because it is all included in the price. Choosing the cheapest food, whether in the restaurant or the supermarket, even if it isn't what you want. Depriving yourself because it's too expensive, even when you know you could afford it financially;

♦ Fear of displeasing. Inability to say no to someone who offers you something to eat or drink, while it was not initially your intention to have anything.

♦ Afraid of letting on that you don't like a certain food once you have tasted it;

♦ Fear of judgment. Doing what others are doing, out of fear of what they will think or say about you;

♦ Fear of the consequences, of being sick if you don't eat. Eating out of obligation, without enjoyment, only to nourish your body.

You are motivated by *HABIT* when:

♦ You often or always eat the same thing. For instance, 2 slices of toast with peanut butter for breakfast;

♦ You often or always eat at the same time;

♦ You act according to what you learned in childhood, like eating three meals a day, never skipping breakfast, etc.;

♦ You hesitate or refuse to try new foods because you have never tasted them.

You are motivated by *EMOTION* when:

♦ You know you are not really hungry, but some impulse drives you to eat or drink all the same;

♦ You ask yourself *I wonder what I should have to*

eat? not knowing what food to choose and knowing that you are not eating out of principle or out of habit;

♦ You are angry, frustrated, sad or lonely and you eat or drink for lack of being able to express your feelings in some other way at that moment.

You are motivated by *GOURMANDISE* when you are influenced by one or more of your five senses:

♦ You eat or drink because it smells good;

♦ You can't stop because it's just so good;

♦ You are attracted by a certain food just because you see it, while a few minutes earlier, you hadn't even thought about it;

♦ You cannot keep from sampling a tray you happen to lay eyes on;

♦ You want to eat the same thing as the person next to you;

♦ You are attracted by a food after touching or smelling it – you like its texture or its aroma – like popcorn at the movie theatre;

♦ When you let yourself be influenced by what you hear, for example, a restaurant waiter giving a mouth-watering description of an item on the menu.

You are motivated by the need to *REWARD* yourself when:

♦ You have just finished a task you are very proud of and so, you feel like having something to eat or drink, knowing very well that you do not need it at that moment;

♦ You have overstepped your limits, having worked relentlessly without taking any time out, and you think that eating will help you to relax;

♦ You feel frustrated because no one is paying you any compliments and so, in the circumstances, you eat indiscriminately. (This situation could also fit in the *EMOTIONS* column).

You are motivated by *LAZINESS* when:

♦ You accept what someone else decides to cook for you rather than have to prepare something yourself;

♦ You are home alone and you decide on a dish that doesn't require any preparation;

♦ You decide not to eat rather than have to fix yourself something;

♦ You buy a pre-cooked or frozen dinner when you leave work, to eat when you get home.

I want to remind you that it is possible to drink something for several of the same reasons contained in the six motivations above, even though only the word "eat" is used with them. As soon as you ask yourself, *What should I drink?* it is important to keep in mind that water is what your body needs. So, every time you drink something else, you must note it down in one of the six columns.

Likewise, you may have to put a checkmark in more than one of the six columns for the same food, for example, eating candy out of emotion as well as for a reward.

A small piece of advice for the perfectionist

It is important not to get stressed out about wanting to complete this journal PERFECTLY. It may be that on several occasions you wonder in which column to put your checkmark. Actually, it doesn't matter a whole lot if it's not in the right box. The main purpose of keeping this journal is to allow yourself to look back over your day and get to know yourself better. Know that this goal has already been achieved as soon as you start taking the time to make your entries and maintain the right motivation.

Interpreting the six motivations

Now, here is the way to interpret the results.

EATING OUT OF PRINCIPLE OR HABIT means that you allow yourself, generally speaking, to be too **controlled or manipulated by your beliefs** in life. Beliefs come mainly from your education and what you learned in childhood and adolescence. It is the past that is directing your life. There are several fears preventing you from listening to your intuition, listening to your genuine needs. Consequently, you must surely be missing out on numerous interesting opportunities. Moreover, it is very probable that you are among those who resist new ideas or suggestions that others offer.

In summary, the person who does not take the time to ask themselves whether they are hungry and who eats on principle or from habit, is a person who lets themselves be directed by the notion of good/evil, supposed to/not sup-

203

posed to, right/wrong. It is their ego that is controlling their stomach. This type of person also finds it hard to enjoy themselves or to taste the pleasures of life, believing it is wrong to do so before all the chores are done. This person might also believe that pleasing others must come before pleasing themselves. This is often the kind of person who, when they are in a store will buy according to the price of an item instead of buying what they would really like at that moment.

EATING OUT OF EMOTION means that you are experiencing a lot more emotion – consciously or not – than you would like to admit. You are someone who tries to block out what you feel. You might be experiencing anger, frustration, disappointment, sadness or loneliness, etc., but you try as much as possible to avoid going too deep and feeling the pain associated with these emotions. It is a method many people use, believing they will suffer less that way. It is important to remember that when you experience emotions, the implication is that you have many expectations. You anticipate, rightly or wrongly, that others will show you love and affection in the way you want them to. Since no one is responsible for the happiness of others, all the times that your expectations are not met, you try to fill this inner void with some kind of substance (a food or beverage). *A priori*, we often have strong emotional reactions when we confuse LOVING and PLEASING.

EATING OUT OF GOURMANDISE means that your senses are not satisfied psychologically and that, generally, you allow yourself to be influenced by them in your life. That is to say, you are influenced by what you see, hear and sense from others. Most of the time, this is due to the fact that you feel responsible for the happiness of others. You must often feel obliged to do something for people in difficulty. Know that those who feel they are responsible for the good fortune or misfortune of others often experience guilt and this is reflected in the way they eat, which is according to the degree of guilt they feel toward others. Furthermore, it is quite likely that you have trouble allowing those you love to make their own choices, especially when you do not agree with them. **Your happiness depends on the happiness of others and this creates an emptiness in your heart that you try to fill with food, instead of learning to fill it by meeting your true needs.**

EATING AS A REWARD means you are someone who asks too much of yourself, often going beyond your limits. You are possibly perfectionist by nature and you wait until you have done or achieved something extraordinary before rewarding yourself. It would appear you often expect others to appreciate you, congratulate you and pay you compliments. There is no one on earth whose job it is to ensure the happiness of others. So, most of us experience disappointment, even bitterness, when our expectations are not met.

EATING OUT OF LAZINESS means that you are probably more dependent on others than you think. When you are in the presence of those you love, you must be a different person than when you are alone. You must find yourself acting according to their choices. It means you do not believe you are important enough. The presence of others brings you this false sense of importance. You do not believe sufficiently in your worth as a person to take the time to listen to your needs. You may also find that when someone else fixes you something good to eat, you have the impression of receiving some form of your mother's love, bringing to mind that happiness or the lack of it.

Conclusion

I suggest that you take stock at the end of each week to obtain a better picture of what is going on in your life. At the end of a week, you will be more aware of what is influencing your life most at present. You will observe what factors most prompt you to eat when you are not listening to your needs. For more details, you can reread Chapter Four.

A FINAL REMINDER... When you discover that you have not listened to your needs very much, as you fill in your journal, take care not to blame yourself. The main objective of this exercise is to know yourself better and to let go of control. So give yourself the right to not always be acting in accordance with your needs or preferences, rather than add yet another stress to your life!

I wish from the bottom of my heart that your decision to complete your daily journal for a period of at least three months will prove very beneficial to you and that in learning to love yourself more, you will discover the marvellous person that you are. Remember the triangle of love. **The more you love yourself, the more you receive love from others and the easier it is for you to love others.**

You may have read this book all in one stretch, without taking into account the suggestions made. The subject of food touches several chords in us, since eating is both a social and an individual event. I recognize therefore that this work may at times shake certain beliefs or habits. However, the fact that you are holding this book in your hands means you are a perfect candidate to set out on this personal journey... so, let me suggest to you that you reread this book and put into practice the suggestions it contains.

Daily **FOOD** Journal

Week of:_____

	Hour	Food and/or beverage	Hungry	Not hungry	Eat as needed	Eat on principle	Eat from habit	Eat out of emotion	Eat out of gourmandise	Eat for a reward	Eat out of laziness	Link
Jour 1 :___												
Jour 2 :___												
Jour 3 :___												

Thank you, my body, for what you have helped me discover today
I know myself a little better each day and I accept myself as I am

	Hour	Food and/or beverage	Hungry	Not hungry	As needed	Principle	Habit	Emotion	Gourmandise	Reward	Laziness	Link
Jour 4 :												
Jour 5 :												
Jour 6 :												
Jour 7 :												

Thank you, my body, for what you have helped me discover today.
I know myself a little better each day and I accept myself as I am.

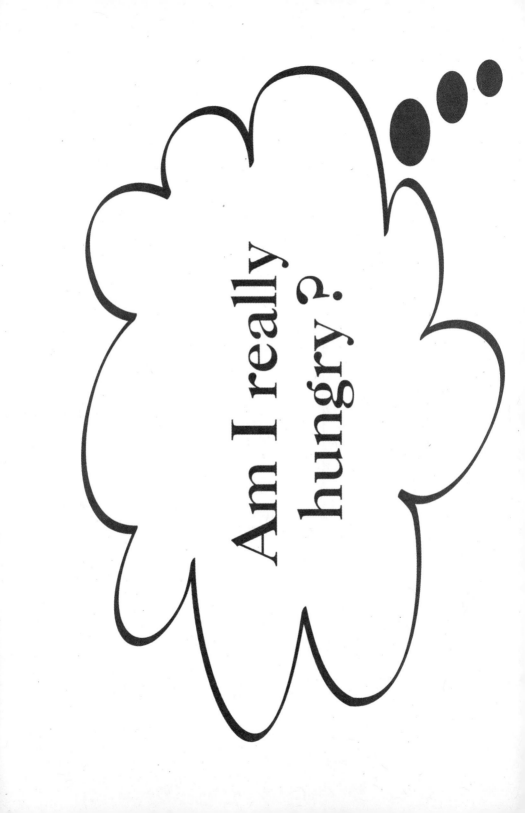

If you would like to receive information about future books by Lise Bourbeau, send us your contact information at…

by e-mail   info@leseditionsetc.com

by fax   450 431 0991

by mail   Les Editions ETC
             1102 Boulevard La Salette
             St-Jérôme (Québec)
             J5L 2J7 CANADA

Who wants to enjoy life?

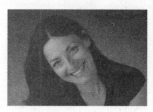

The dynamic and powerful teachings of the "Listen to Your Body" workshop are aimed at all people who are interested in **enjoying their life**. For the past 25 years, this workshop has provided participants with a vital source of knowledge as well as a solid foundation for being in harmony with themselves. Year after year, the startling results and enriching transformations achieved by over 40,000 people who have attended this workshop are truly astounding. **Those who read her books were surprised to see how much further the workshop brought them.**

Improve the quality of your life in just 2 days!

- ► Are you happy?
- ► Do you often feel guilty?
- ► Is disappointment part of your life?
- ► Do you get along with people easily?
- ► Are you full of energy?
- ► Do you have the life you want?
- ► Is it difficult for you to say no?
- ► Do you need to be perfect before loving yourself?

Come and see how our workshop can help you!

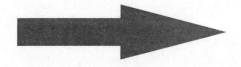

Stop putting up with your problems!

Thanks to this workshop, thousands of people are no longer putting up with life - they are living it! They have regained control over their lives and are using the wealth of personal power within them to create the lives they really want. The rewards are far greater than could be imagined.

The "Listen to Your Body" workshop has tangible effects at all levels: physical, emotional, mental and spiritual.

What do people think?

"Thanks for filling my heart and giving me new tools!"

"Thank you so much for a wonderful weekend. I look forward to growing!"

"It has been a delight and an honor to spend this time with you. Thank you for all the insights, the education and the fun! I wish you all the best."

"It has been a wonderful experience!"

"Thank you for sharing your wisdom... you inspire me."

"Thanks for a great weekend. The info will last a lifetime and improve it as I walk the path."

"Thank you for the light you shone on my path. The future reserves many nice surprises and I have the impression that your light will be part of it."

Visit our website or call us

To find out when and where the next workshop will be held.

1-888-437-8382 or 450-431-5336
www.listentoyourbody.net

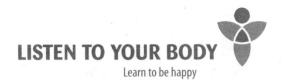

LISTEN TO YOUR BODY

Learn to be happy

Don't miss a thing!

Subscribe today
to receive our
bi-monthly
newsletter
including advice
from Lise

It's easy!

Visit our website
and fill in the
subscription
window on our
home page

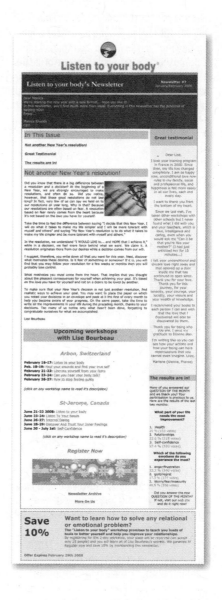

www.listentoyourbody.net

Books from the same author

Listen to your best friend on Earth, your body

LISE BOURBEAU takes you by the hand and, step by step, leads you beyond "packing your own parachute", to taking that step back into the clear, refreshing stream of life that flows from the Universal Source. She gives you the tools, not only to fix what is wrong in your life, but to build a solid foundation for your inner house - a foundation that extends as far as the global village. In this book, she helps you build an intimate, rewarding and powerful relationship with the most important person in your life - yourself.

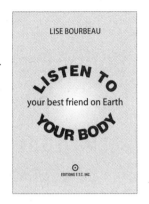

Your body's telling you: Love yourself!

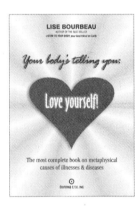

Lise Bourbeau has compiled 20 years of research in the field of metaphysics and it's physical manifestations in the body and brought it all to the forefront in this user-friendly reference guide, Your body's telling you: Love yourself! Since 1982, she has worked successfully with over 15,000 people, helping them to unearth the underlying causes of specific illnesses and diseases.

"I am certain that any physical problem is simply the outward manifestation of dis-ease on psychological and/or emotional levels. The physical body is responding to this imbalance and warning of the need to return to the path of love and harmony."

Cover to cover, the reader discovers a most powerful tool, as he becomes his own healer. The reference material, a comprehensive guide to the causes of over 500 illnesses and diseases, is a succinct and visionary work that is truly and literally a labor of love.

Heal your wounds and find your true self

Do you sometimes feel that you are going around in circles in your personal growth? Do you occasionally see a problem re-emerge, thinking you had solved it? Perhaps it's because you're not looking in the right place.

This new book by Lise Bourbeau, as concrete as her others, demonstrates that all problems, whether physical, emotional or mental, stem from five important wounds: *rejection, abandonment, humiliation, betrayal* and *injustice*. This book contains detailed descriptions of these wounds and of the masks we've developed to hide them.

This book will allow you to set off on the path that leads to complete healing, the path that leads to your ultimate goal: your true self.

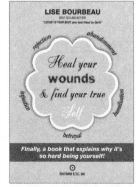

4 ways to order

TITLE	QTY.	TOTAL
	SUB-TOTAL	
	SHIPPING	
	TOTAL	

info@listentoyourbody.net

450-431-0991

ECOUTE TON CORPS
1102 La Salette Blv
St-Jerome (Quebec)
J5L 2J7   CANADA

**1-800-361-3834
or 450-431-5336**

SHIPPING & HANDLING FEES
CANADA: 8.50$can
US: 10$can
INTERNATIONAL: contact us

VISA ☐   Number: ☐☐☐☐☐☐☐☐☐☐☐☐☐☐☐☐☐☐☐   Exp.: ☐☐ / ☐☐
                                                                   month   year

MasterCard ☐   Cardholder's name: _____

Signature: _____

☐ **CANADIAN MONEY ORDER made out to ECOUTE TON CORPS**

Name: _____

Address: _____

City/Town: _____   Zip code: _____

Telephone #: (_____) _____